Pain Relief in Labour

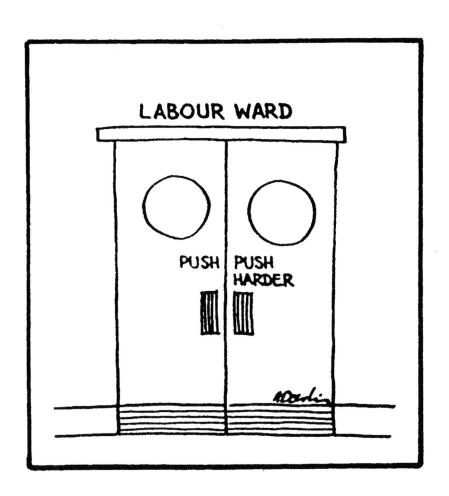

Pain Relief in Labour

by

Robin Russell
Jackie Porter
Mark Scrutton

Edited by
Felicity Reynolds

BMJ
Publishing
Group

© BMJ Publishing Group 1997

First published in 1997
by the BMJ Publishing Group, BMA House, Tavistock Square,
London WC1H 9JR

British Library Cataloguing in Publication Data

A catalogue record for this book is available from the
British Library

ISBN 0-7279-1009-4

Typeset, printed and bound in Great Britain by
Latimer Trend & Company Ltd, Plymouth

Contents

Contributors

Jackie Porter MB BS, FRCA
One-time research fellow, Anaesthetic Unit (UMDS), St Thomas's Hospital; currently specialist registrar, St Thomas' Hospital, London

Felicity Reynolds MD, FRCA, FRCOG
Emeritus Professor of Obstetric Anaesthesia (UMDS), St Thomas's Hospital, London

Robin Russell MB BS, MD, FRCA
One-time research fellow, Anaesthetic Unit (UMDS), St Thomas's Hospital; currently Consultant Anaesthetist, John Radcliffe Hospital, Oxford

Mark Scrutton MB BS, FRCA
One-time research fellow, Anaesthetic Unit (UMDS), St Thomas's Hospital; currently specialist registrar, St Thomas's Hospital, London

Acknowledgements

We thank *Private Eye* for permission to use the frontispiece. The cartoon on page 158 is by Stavros Prineas and first appeared in the *International Journal of Obstetric Anesthesia*, 1996;5:140. The cartoon on page 180 is from an idea by Colm Lanigan, generated by Tove Tunnard. The cartoon on page 231 is copyright of Nash Enterprises, 1994. The cartoon on page 237 is by Felicity Reynolds. The cartoon character on page 241 was generated by Tove Tunnard.

Preface

The aim of this book is to bring under one umbrella such different types of analgesia as have been studied for use in labour. Unfortunately, while the usual methods of search for information yield a copious amount relating to epidural and systemic analgesia, little is to be found on non-pharmacological methods. Such sources of information as exist relating to the various alternative approaches to pain relief, rarely provide reliable evidence for their efficacy or side effects in the form of randomised trials.[1] This is a shame because mothers deserve to be given well-founded information rather than anecdote, about all the techniques they may have recommended to them. Moreover, in writing this book we are in danger of being accused of bias in allotting what might seem a disproportionate amount of space to regional analgesia. In fact, if the number of pages is related to the volume of reliable source material, we find regional analgesia is actually under-represented. It would be both tedious and inappropriate to provide a completely comprehensive review of the literature on regional analgesia in labour.

We hope, nevertheless, that the balance of this book may serve to broaden the knowledge base of our anaesthetic colleagues while also providing some practical guidance in the pursuit of their own particular skills. We hope that midwives and obstetricians may derive benefit from this text; though it is written by anaesthetists, we have striven to maintain objectivity and to tell a balanced story.

We have not included a section on anaesthesia in obstetrics as an ample bibliography now exists on this topic. Our intention was to provide a more comprehensive and practical account of pain relief than is found in the existing texts on the subject of obstetric anaesthesia.

FELICITY REYNOLDS

Reference

1 Chalmers I. Scientific inquiry and authoritarianism in perinatal care and education. *Birth* 1983;**10**:151–64.

1: Introduction: Labour pain and analgesia

Introduction

The control of pain should form an integral part of the management of labour, yet pain relief in labour is a surprisingly controversial subject in the UK; among both carers and consumers there are those who have quite erroneous views of the risks of effective pain relief while being ignorant of the benefits.

Pregnant women have a right to basic information about pain and its relief in labour, as well as other aspects of their care. It is therefore important that all those involved, whether general practitioner, midwife, obstetrician or anaesthetist, should be well informed about all types of pain relief that are available. Midwives, who observe all sorts of mothers using many methods of pain relief, certainly have the broadest view, so it is appropriate that they most commonly handle mothers' questions during pregnancy. Yet they are sometimes unaware of the full story, while anaesthetists, who may be more or less well informed about regional analgesia, are commonly ignorant of other forms of pain relief. We have therefore tried to bring together such of the available information as is reliable, on most types of pain relief, in order to allow carers to broaden their knowledge base and to be better able to answer the mothers' questions. Yet information that is given to mothers must be tempered by a thorough knowledge of local practice. It is useless to tell a mother how wonderful the effects of reflexology can be if there is no reflexologist available to train her. Similarly, it is inappropriate to tell her that the only reliable form of pain relief is epidural analgesia if an epiduralist is available from 10·00 to 4·00 on Tuesdays and Thursdays only *or* if the local service is of poor quality and, for example, the accidental dural puncture rate exceeds 1%.

The severity of labour pain

Although the severity of pain varies greatly among women in labour, numerous studies demonstrate quite consistently that if women are asked during or very shortly after labour to score their labour pain most rate it as severe while few have little or no pain.[1-4] In a survey in London, UK,[5] only 2% of women questioned one or two days postpartum reported a painless labour. In one Swedish survey, even when questioned one or two days postpartum 35% of women recollected intolerable pain, 37% severe and 28% moderate.[4] These workers found that late antenatal care, unwanted pregnancy, anxiety, and poor education were associated with an increase in the level of reported pain. In a Finnish survey of 833 parturients[6] 4% reported only mild pain, and after delivery 60% of them said that the pain was severe or intolerable. Using the McGill Pain Questionnaire Melzack *et al* in Montreal, Canada, found that labour pain usually rated a high score particularly among primiparae, those with a history of dysmenorrhoea and those of low socio-economic status.[1] Primiparae who had attended prepared childbirth classes reported less pain than those who had not, though more than 80% requested epidurals in both groups. Davenport-Slack and Boylan[7] pointed out that preparation for childbirth can provide a model for good behaviour rather than a means of reducing pain. Good training during pregnancy helps to allay a mother's fear and anxiety, hence when faced with severe pain she may behave more calmly, emphasising the value of honesty in preparation for childbirth. The effect of psychological preparation for childbirth on the experience of labour pain is discussed more fully in Chapter 2.

Pain during labour of spontaneous onset tends to build up gradually, whereas when labour is induced and accelerated artificially the initial pain may be severe and hence more difficult to bear. A national survey conducted by the UK National Birthday Trust (NBT) in 1990 showed the use of epidural analgesia in induced labour to be double that in spontaneous.[8] Although primiparae are sometimes reported to experience more pain than multiparae, this is almost certainly related in part to the length of time for which they suffer pain. Pain during a multiparous short, strong labour can indeed be severe, but may be better tolerated because more quickly over, and hence more easily forgotten. Data from the NBT survey[8] showed clearly that the need for effective pain relief in the form of epidural analgesia increases with the length of labour (Figure 1.1).

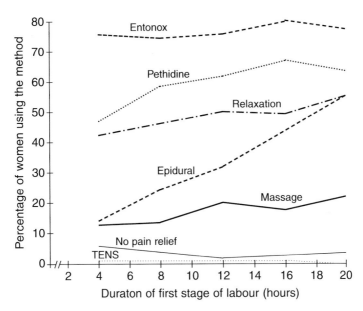

FIGURE 1.1—*All methods of analgesia used by nulliparous women according to duration of labour. (From Chamberlain* et al[8] *by permission of the authors and publisher)*

Pain cannot be judged by an onlooker since individuals vary greatly in their response to pain, and moreover observers may mistake sedation for analgesia. This is a well-recognised phenomenon where the effect of pethidine is concerned.[8] Also pain rated after the event becomes progressively more inaccurate.[9] Memories of pain fade consistently.[8-11] One study comparing pain recorded during labour with that recollected subsequently showed that by the second day recollected pain had reduced to 50%.[10] In general the more severe the pain the more its memory is obliterated in later months. This amnesia was highlighted by Morgan et al,[11] who showed that among mothers who had reported severe labour pain, more than 90% had forgotten its severity 3 months later, when they viewed the experience with satisfaction.

Why then this amnesia for the pain of labour? The phenomenon of transmarginal inhibition can cause amnesia towards stressful events – Nature's way of protecting the psyche. This effect is probably enhanced by the euphoria engendered at the birth of a live baby. If, however, the outcome is stillbirth the memory of a painful labour and delivery may be less likely to fade.

Those who remember experiencing a tolerable labour in which they required little or no analgesia should bear in mind that some of the pain

3

will certainly have been blotted out while a relatively painless labour is the exception rather than the rule. Such women should be counted lucky; the majority are not so fortunate. Parturients who also take a professional interest in labour need to make a mental or an actual note about their pain during or shortly after their experience if they wish to recall it accurately. Those who have done so can bear witness that though their approach may have been calm, well-informed, unafraid and relaxed, they could still experience excruciating pain.

The value of pain relief

If pain is so quickly forgotten and the greater the pain the greater the postnatal euphoria, then why use artificial means to treat it? First, though pain may be quickly forgotten this does not make it any more tolerable at the time; it is therefore only humane to attempt to relieve it. Secondly, though anxiety may be believed to exacerbate pain, relieving pain can quite dramatically reduce a mother's anxiety. Thirdly, the pain of labour represents severe physiological stress[12] which can result in maternal metabolic acidosis and hormone imbalance including catecholamine release. Stimulation of α-receptors causes vasoconstriction which may affect the maternal blood supply to the placenta while β stimulation may prolong labour.[13,14] These represent adverse effects not only for the mother but also for the baby[12-17] (Figure 1.2) and can be corrected by the use of epidural analgesia.

Aspects of neuroanatomy, physiology and pharmacology relevant to pain and its relief in labour are to be found in Chapter 3 on physical methods of pain relief and Chapter 7, which explores the basic sciences of regional analgesia.

Labour analgesia in the Western world in perspective

Few national surveys of pain and its relief in labour have been carried out. A summary of the results of a selection of them[3,8,18-20] is given in Table 1.1. Though much has been spoken and written in the lay press about various non-pharmacological methods of pain relief, in practice most women also use some form of pharmacological analgesia.[8] In many countries some form of inhalational analgesia is used, as are narcotics (mostly commonly pethidine but occasionally morphine or various synthetic partial opioid agonists), while regional analgesia is commonly used in between 20 and 30% of women. The history of these different types of analgesia is given in each of the relevant chapters.

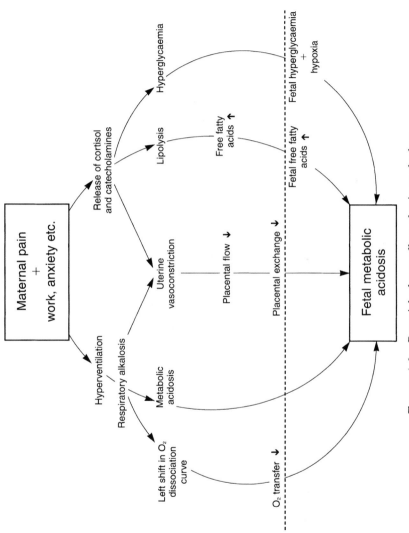

FIGURE 1.2—*Potential adverse effects of pain on the fetus*

TABLE 1.1—*Estimated percentage overall use of different methods of analgesia, derived from national surveys*

	USA 1981	USA 1992	Sweden 1983–6	Finland 1991	UK 1990
Number of deliveries surveyed	?	?	335 207	890	12 467
No analgesia	32	22	1·5	2·4	8·3
Opioid	49	54	49	19	38
Inhalational	n/k	n/k	n/k	56	>60
Paracervical block	0	0	12	19	0
Epidural/spinal	16	33	16	14	20

No analgesia may include "non-pharmacological".
n/k, not known.
USA 1981: survey of 1200 hospitals[18]; 1992: survey of 1400 hospitals[19]
Sweden 1983–6: national survey, vaginal deliveries only[20]
Finland 1991: national survey, 1 week[3]
UK 1990: national survey, 1 week[8]

With the decline of paternalistic medicine it is considered politically correct to pay attention to women's views. Though it is hard to argue with this concept, it is equally inappropriate to be too readily swayed by consumer movements that may not necessarily be evidence-based. A glance at the history of pain relief in labour during this century lends support to this seemingly heretical view.

Herbs of various kinds have been used for many centuries to relieve labour pain, but the subject first attracted major attention in the nineteenth century when volatile anaesthetics such as ether and chloroform, which were probably far more effective, were introduced. The controversy surrounding this is well known, particularly for its lack of materialist logic. Now more frequently forgotten is the probably much more dangerous and considerably less logical era of twilight sleep, a technique originating in Germany that swept America at the start of this century.[21] The impetus was provided by consumers with, to do it credit, some resistance from the medical profession. A state of delirium and amnesia rather than analgesia was created which could be harmful to both mother and baby. Since it was recognised that the technique required careful monitoring there was a consumer-led demand for hospital rather than home delivery. A similar move towards hospital delivery has been seen during this century in the UK. During the 1970s home delivery, once the norm, fell below 10% and it is currently 1–2%. This trend has occurred at a time of dramatic improvement in maternal and perinatal mortality, and the present campaign to de-medicalise childbirth and emphasise home birth as a reasonable choice is as devoid of supporting evidence as was twilight sleep.

A move towards more so-called natural childbirth was probably an appropriate reaction to the overuse of sedation in hospitals. It had its modern origins in the movement largely pioneered by Grantly Dick Read in the 1930s. Remarkable claims have been made for natural childbirth techniques,[22] that they reduce the incidence of many complications (see Chapter 2), but these claims are not based on good evidence. They stem from anecdote rather than randomised controlled trial. To conduct a randomised trial, however, would hardly be ethical, since we already have overwhelming evidence on a global scale of the outcome of truly natural childbirth without interference. In areas where few of the community have access to skilled medical assistance, such as parts of the Indian subcontinent and particularly rural Africa, childbirth is consistently natural. The image of a mother bringing her baby into the world with little fuss in such circumstances is misleading in the extreme. Maternal mortality in these parts may be as high as 1 in 200 and perinatal mortality 1 in 10.[23] Such statistics also pertained in the Western world before 1935,[24] but nowadays with maternal mortality rates in the developed world less than 1 in 10 000 and perinatal mortality less than 1 in 100, we expect to improve on nature.

Homeopathy, acupuncture and hypnosis are used by a combined total of fewer than 0·5% of women in the UK.[8] TENS is much more widely available in Britain and more frequently used, but although harmless, it

TABLE 1.2—*Antenatal class attended and principal type of pain relief planned, used and planned next time (n = 2841)*

Type of class (% of women attending)		Non-pharm. (%)	TENS (%)	Nitrous oxide (%)	Pethidine (%)	Epidural (%)
Health	Planned	10·5	2·2	35·6	34·8	16·9
Centre	Used	6·6	0·8	27·7	42·7	22·2
(34%)	Next	5·2	1·4	26·1	36·1	31·3
Hospital	Planned	10·2	2·6	35·2	33·4	18·6
(24%)	Used	5·6	1·2	28·9	37·6	26·6
	Next	5·2	1·3	27·0	29·5	37·0
NCT	Planned	11·4	10·3	47·6	15·1	15·7
(4%)	Used	13·0	5·4	37·8	21·1	22·7
	Next	10·8	4·9	38·9	14·6	30·8
All attending	Planned	10·4	3·3	36·2	33·0	17·5
classes	Used	6·6	1·2	28·8	39·3	23·9
(63%)[a]	Next	5·6	1·6	27·8	32·3	33·5

[a]1% of women surveyed attended types of classes other than those listed here.
Non-pharm., non-pharmacological methods
TENS, transcutaneous electrical nerve stimulation
NCT, National Childbirth Trust

Data from NBT survey[8]

has often given rise to disappointment, many women turning with relief to nitrous oxide or epidural analgesia.[8] It must surely be an expensive but labour-saving alternative to rubbing the back. In some centres insufficient emphasis may be placed on training a partner to perform this function. Among the various opioid analgesics, pethidine is widely used and available in virtually all obstetric units. In the NBT survey it was rated by mothers as little better than TENS, while midwives over-rated its value.[8]

The method of analgesia planned and used differed slightly depending upon the type of antenatal class attended (Table 1.2): those attending National Childbirth Trust (NCT) classes were more likely to plan and use TENS and less likely to plan or use pethidine than those attending NHS classes, whether at a health centre or in a hospital.

Nitrous oxide was in all groups the most used form of analgesia (Figure 1.1). About 75% of women probably had it at some time during their labour and indeed it was the most popular method among women who had attended NCT classes. Extensive use of nitrous oxide in the UK may relate in part to its availability in the form of Entonox, which is highly convenient and safe. Although in 1974 Holdcroft and Morgan[5] had demonstrated the clear superiority of nitrous oxide over pethidine for analgesia in labour, this fact evidently came as a surprise to the organisers and compilers of the NBT survey, who had regarded pethidine as a more powerful analgesic than nitrous oxide. It cannot be too strongly emphasised that this is not the case.

Epidural analgesia

Epidural analgesia is not universally available in the UK. It is an expensive and time-consuming option and it is impossible and indeed unsafe to provide it in smaller units. According to the NBT survey, however, failure to provide epidural analgesia was the single most frequent cause of anxiety and disappointment among labouring women.[8] Some women reported reluctance among midwives to provide it while others felt they had been conditioned to believe they would not require it and wished they had been prepared more realistically. The longer the labour lasted, however, the more likely the woman would be to be given her epidural in the end (Figure 1.1). Although among those attending antenatal classes only 17% stated that they had intended to have epidural analgesia, 24% actually required it. Moreover 33% stated they planned to have epidural analgesia next time as did 76% of women replying to a later questionnaire. This is evidence of inappropriate preparation for childbirth; surely women should be warned that they are more likely to need epidural analgesia for the first than for a

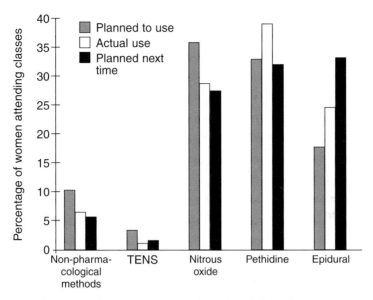

FIGURE 1.3—*Percentage of women who planned, used and planned to use next time the different methods of pain relief. Data from the NBT survey (see Table 1.2)*[8]

subsequent labour. Such apparent escalation in demand is not seen for other types of pain relief (Figure 1.3).

Though epidural rates in Western countries may appear to be roughly similar (Table 1.1), the similarities conceal wide differences in rates between hospitals.[8,20,25] These differences appear to be dictated more by local fashion than by medical need; availability appears to condition a mother's expectations. Are these the best reasons to provide epidural analgesia? There are many reasons outlined in Chapter 8 why effective regional analgesia should be used in high-risk obstetrics but units without expertise in the field will inevitably provide a second-rate service when it is needed.

A survey carried out for the five years 1988–92 in the South East Thames Region[25] demonstrated some interesting anomalies. While the average epidural rate in Maidstone was about 10%, that in the next-door district of Pembury was 24%. Both hospitals serve wealthy country towns and rural communities. Nearer to London the epidural rate in Sidcup was around 14% and in next-door Farnborough, 27%. In the inner city the communities are served by university teaching hospitals, and while the neighbourhoods are all universally poor, with a heavy load of high-risk obstetrics, epidural rates are between 17 and 27% in three of the hospitals but over 40% in the fourth. In the latter hospital, although only 10–12% of women expecting their first babies planned to request epidural analgesia, more than 60% actually did so when they experienced labour. A study among these women found that they did not so much under-estimate the pain of labour as over-estimate their own capacity to cope with it.[26] A dedicated epidural service upon which the midwives felt they could rely meant that these women could be encouraged to exercise a woman's inalienable privilege to change her mind.

Epidural analgesia is both the hero and the villain of pain relief in labour. The hero because, as women consistently showed in the NBT[8] and other surveys,[6,9] it is the only reliable means of providing effective analgesia in labour. The villain because without appropriate training and skills there is tremendous scope for mismanagement and hence dissatisfaction. It is to be hoped that its capacity to do serious damage is reducing with improvements in technique. Regrettably, however, there are insufficient trained anaesthetists in the UK and many countries to provide an efficient epidural service universally. The recent closure of small units was helpful, but if this trend goes into reverse, one can foresee a further decline in services.

An advantage of the centralised approach to obstetric care is that it increases the range of services that can be made available to a mother. A dedicated obstetric anaesthesia service is one such. To have a dedicated anaesthetist to provide epidural analgesia has the advantage that this anaesthetist is more likely to be available in the event of catastrophe, to provide anaesthesia for emergency caesarean section or resuscitation of the mother. Moreover, with a well-run service obstetric disasters are more likely to make calls upon the anaesthetist than are epidural catastrophes. Most airline passengers probably believe that the main purpose of the cabin crew is to provide food and drink and general comfort, whereas in truth their prime function is to shepherd passengers off the aeroplane in the event of a disaster. Similarly anaesthetists may be perceived as only providing the frills in childbirth but such a requirement is likely to ensure their immediate presence to fulfil their essential emergency role. A move back towards more community based units and even home delivery is believed to foster maternal choice. A mother's choice, let alone her safety, is not, however, enhanced by denying her the full range of options for care in labour.

Who should inform the mother about pain and methods of analgesia?

Information may come not only from antenatal classes but also from friends and relations, books, videos and by questioning staff at clinics. Regrettably in many centres only the minority of women attend antenatal classes and those tend to be the ones who also read books and become generally informed. It is important therefore that every brief encounter at an antenatal clinic should be used to ensure the spread of information among the less well-motivated women. Every expectant mother should also be given a leaflet bearing essential information about the types of pain relief available locally. There is otherwise a danger that women acquire information from individuals who lack a breadth of knowledge. The best teachers are those who have seen countless women in labour rather than those who speak from personal experience. Individual experience is unreliable, first because labour is infinitely variable and secondly, the pain of labour, particularly if severe, is remarkably soon forgotten.[11] Regrettably, among the lay, those most eager to inform and even to conduct antenatal classes are often women who have been fortunate enough to have relatively easy labours or labours that, though severely painful, ended in a relatively swift normal delivery. In such circumstances the adverse aspect of the experience is soon forgotten in the satisfaction of a new baby with its accompanying euphoriant effect.

Such lay individuals, with the best of intentions, may tell mothers that labour can be relatively trouble-free provided interference is avoided. This rather puts the cart before the horse and can lead a mother to feel resentful when she finds that labour is indeed painful and that intervention is required. She may also erroneously feel guilt and a sense of failure when she needs pain relief: not an ideal frame of mind in which to undergo parturition. A woman who has appropriate expectations and trusts her carers will tend to accept their advice with greater equanimity, hence the sort of tension that can only exacerbate a difficult and long labour is less likely to arise.

At the other extreme anaesthetists are usually inappropriate people to be solely responsible for providing information about pain relief. Most anaesthetists only meet those requiring regional analgesia or anaesthesia. They rarely see the lucky women who have relatively easy labours or those who manage without their ministrations.

It is clear, therefore, that midwives are the ideal people to inform women about pain and its relief in childbirth, but those midwives not only require continuing experience in the unit in which their mothers are expected to deliver, they must also have the facts at their fingertips. It is inappropriate to suggest to a nullipara that she must decide what type of pain relief she would like to have before the event, without giving her a true picture of what she is likely to encounter. On the other hand, it may also be misleading to suggest a mother should "keep an open mind" without giving her guidance about what is likely to be effective and what not. It is sometimes suggested to a mother that she can *choose* what type of labour to have and

11

whatever type of analgesia she would like. This can be misleading in several ways. Regrettably a mother, particularly a nulliparous woman, cannot *choose* to have a quick easy labour without complications requiring intervention, nor can she *choose* to be able to cope with the pain unaided. Birth plans can be misleading in this respect. Also, as is pointed out above, obstetric units vary greatly in the types of analgesia that they can provide universally and skilfully.

Where an efficient epidural service is available it is not necessary to hoodwink a mother that labour is unlikely to be painful. It is better she is warned to expect severe pain but reassured that it is possible to alleviate it. Then if she finds herself to be among the lucky few who do not experience severe pain, she can only be thankful. Even where there is no full epidural service it is probably as well to make it clear that labour is likely to be painful – a common complaint among mothers surveyed after parturition is that they were never warned what it would be like.[8] They can at least be taught how best to cope. If pain is anticipated, when it occurs it is less likely to engender fear.

The role of the anaesthetist

Clearly anaesthetists do have a role in antenatal preparation and should attend antenatal classes and be prepared to answer mothers' questions about methods of analgesia. Videos about regional analgesia may also be helpful as they may give mothers a clearer picture of what they are likely to encounter. Any video that is to be used should be vetted carefully by both midwife and anaesthetist to see where the procedures that are portrayed differ from local practices.

A close liaison between anaesthetists, midwives and obstetricians in relation to antenatal care and preparation has another use. Nowadays many women with serious chronic diseases may become pregnant. It is important that these women should be assessed antenatally by a senior anaesthetist and that a management plan for delivery be made before the onset of labour. Good communication between obstetrician, midwife, physician, haematologist and any other relevant specialist can help the anaesthetist in high-risk pregnancy. It is regrettably easy for serious illness, deformity or disability to be overlooked in antenatal clinics and an anaesthetist who maintains good contact can usefully act as liaison physician for the obstetrician. Because it is usually impossible for an anaesthetist to see every woman who books for delivery in an obstetric unit during pregnancy, he/she is dependent on referrals from obstetricians and increasingly from midwives and general practitioners. It is therefore useful to provide all those conducting antenatal clinics with checklists that can help to point the way to identify those women who present a risk from the anaesthetic point of view.

References

1 Melzack R, Taenzer P, Feldman P, Finch RA. Labour is still painful after prepared childbirth training. *Can Med Assoc J* 1981;**125**:357–63.
2 Melzack R, Kinch R, Dobkin P, Lebrun M, Taenzer P. Severity of labour pain: influence of physical as well as psychological values. *Can Med Assoc J* 1984;**130**:579–84.
3 Kangas-Saarela T, Kangas-Karki T. Pain and pain relief in labour: parturients' experiences. *Int J Obstet Anesth* 1994;**3**:67–74.
4 Nettelbladt P, Fagerstrom C-F, Uddenberg N. The significance of reported childbirth pain. *J Psychosom Res* 1976;**20**:215–21.
5 Holdcroft A, Morgan M. An assessment of the analgesic effect in labour of pethidine and 50 per cent nitrous oxide in oxygen (Entonox). *J Obstet Gynaecol Br Commonw* 1974;**81**: 603–7.
6 Ranta P, Jouppila P, Spalding M, Kangas-Saarela T, Hollmen A, Jouppila R. Parturients' assessment of water blocks, pethidine, nitrous oxide, paracervical and epidural blocks in labour. *Int J Obstet Anesth* 1994;**3**:193–8.
7 Davenport-Slack B, Boylan CH. Psychological correlates of childbirth pain. *Psychosom Med* 1974;**36**:215–23.
8 Chamberlain G, Wraight A, Steer P. *Pain and its relief in childbirth*. (Report of the 1990 NBT Survey.) Edinburgh: Churchill Livingstone, 1993.
9 Robinson JU, Rosen M, Evans JM, Revill SI, David H, Rees GAD. Maternal opinion about analgesia for labour. A controlled trial between epidural block and intramuscular pethidine combined with inhalation. *Anaesthesia* 1980;**35**:1173–81.
10 Norvell KT, Gaston-Johansson F, Fridh G. Rememberance of labor pain: how valid are retrospective pain measurements? *Pain* 1987;**31**:77–86.
11 Morgan BM, Bulpitt CJ, Clifton P, Lewis PJ. Analgesia and satisfaction in childbirth (The Queen Charlotte's 1000 mother survey). *Lancet* 1982;**ii**:808–10.
12 Moore J. The effects of analgesia and anaesthesia on the maternal stress response. In: Reynolds F, ed. *Effects on the baby of maternal analgesia and anaesthesia*. London: WB Saunders, 1993:148–62.
13 Lederman RP, Lederman E, Work BA, McCann DS. The relationship of maternal anxiety, plasma catecholamines, and plasma cortisol to progress in labor. *Am J Obstet Gynecol* 1978;**132**:495–500.
14 Lederman RP, Lederman E, Work BA, McCann DS. Anxiety and epinephrine in multiparous women in labor: relationship to duration of labor and fetal heart rate pattern. *Am J Obstet Gynecol* 1985;**153**:870–7.
15 Rankin JHG, McLaughlin MK. The regulation of the placental blood flow. *J Devel Physiol* 1979;**1**:3–30.
16 Shnider SM, Abboud TK, Artal R. Maternal catecholamines decrease during labor after epidural anesthesia. *Am J Obstet Gynecol* 1983;**147**:13–15.
17 Falconer AD, Powles AB. Plasma noradrenaline levels during labour. *Anaesthesia* 1982; **37**:416–20.
18 Gibbs CP, Krischer J, Peckham BM, Sharp H. Obstetric anesthesia: a national survey. *Anesthesiol* 1986;**65**:298–396.
19 Gibbs CP. Obstetric Anesthesia: USA. Society for Obstetric Anesthesia and Perinatology 28th annual meeting, Tucson, Arizona 1996. Abstract p69.
20 Gerdin E, Cnattingius S. The use of obstetric analgesia in Sweden 1983–1986. *Br J Obstet Gynaecol* 1990;**97**:789–96.
21 Pitcock C de H, Clark RB. From Fanny to Fernand: the development of consumerism in pain control during the birth process. *Am J Obstet Gynecol* 1992;**167**:581–7.
22 Beck NC, Hall D. Natural childbirth. A review and analysis. *Obstet Gynecol* 1978;**52**: 371–9.

13

23 AbouZahr C, Royston E. *Maternal mortality: a global factbook*. Geneva: World Health Organisation, 1991.
24 Department of Health. *Report on Confidential Enquiries into Maternal Deaths in England and Wales 1982–84*. London: HMSO, 1989.
25 Hanson PL, Wolfe CDA. *Perinatal profile: a review of South East Thames perinatal statistics*. South Thames Regional Health Authority, 1995.
26 Reynolds F. Pain relief in labour. *Br J Obstet Gynaecol* 1990;**97**:757–9.

Part One
Non-pharmacological methods

2: Psychological methods of pain relief

Methods of psychological analgesia can be divided into three main categories:

- Natural childbirth – the Read method
- Psychoprophylaxis – the Lamaze technique
- Hypnosis

Proponents of each technique claim the elimination of pain in a high percentage of women without harmful effects to the mother, the baby or the progress of labour, and without the need for chemical analgesia. All require considerable antenatal preparation. Some women still adhere to the traditional teachings of Read and Lamaze, but many forms of preparation include psychological as well as physical elements.

17

Preparation for labour

In its broadest sense, psychological preparation for labour describes a form of antenatal preparation that includes education, distraction and relaxation, designed to reduce pain and to cope with pain in labour. It is generally accepted that the psychological state and antenatal preparation are important determinants of how a woman copes with pain during her labour and how she perceives her labour experience.

Preparation for "natural childbirth"

Natural childbirth was pioneered by a London doctor, Grantly Dick Read. He published a book called *Natural Childbirth*[1] in 1933, which describes his philosophy on coping with labour by natural processes. He believed that through ignorance, prejudice, and misinformation women approached labour with fear, anxiety, and mental tension, all of which gave rise to muscle tension including the myometrium. The result was a poorly dilating cervix, prolonged labour, and pain. Through antenatal education and training Read claimed that fear could be eliminated, labour would be painless, and unnecessary analgesia would be avoided. He believed that women of primitive tribes experienced no pain in labour and pain felt by women in the developed world was purely a result of society-induced expectations, stating "there is no physiologic function in the body which gives rise to pain in the normal course of health", and "for the perfect labour anaesthesia is unnecessary ... there is no pain". He developed a regime of antenatal education and training aimed at creating a state of mind that would prevent the "fear–tension–pain syndrome". His psychotherapeutic training became known as "preparation for natural childbirth". It comprised a series of eight lectures on the anatomy and physiology of pregnancy and labour, and a programme of physical exercises and techniques of muscle relaxation and breathing control for use during labour. Much in advance of his day he also encouraged the partner to be present. Much emphasis was placed on spontaneous vaginal delivery and the avoidance of pharmacological analgesia. He claimed a 95% success rate in reducing the fear and therefore pain of childbirth, although even his supporters doubted this success.

Psychoprophylaxis

Psychoprophylaxis was developed by Velvowski in Russia in 1947 and brought to Western Europe by Dr Ferdinand Lamaze, a French obstetrician, who described it in his book *Painless Childbirth*,[2] published in 1958. It is a method of conditioned reflex training for childbirth, based on the Pavlovian conditioned reflex. Like Read, Velvowski and Lamaze believed that women experienced pain in labour purely because they were conditioned to believe they would. Parturients could be deconditioned and then reconditioned, using positive conditioned reflexes such as breathing exercises and relaxation techniques, to avoid the perception of pain. Thus a uterine contraction could be the signal for the initiation of a new repetitive acquired respiratory reflex. Women are taught to inhale and exhale deeply and slowly at the start of a contraction and then to breathe in a specific shallow pattern during the contraction. This would require intense concentration, sufficient to reduce or eliminate the awareness of labour pain. Essentially this is a form of distraction therapy in which abdominal massage, physical relaxation, breathing exercises and focusing on a specific point in the room all help to block painful stimuli from reaching consciousness. The Russian originators agreed that only a very small percentage of women would feel no pain, yet Lamaze continued to call it "childbirth without pain" and claimed to achieve this for 90% of women.

Antenatal preparation in the 1990s

Preparation for childbirth has become an important part of antenatal care in many maternity centres and the programmes used in most delivery units in the UK have evolved from the teachings of Read and Lamaze. They present a more balanced form of education commonly called "prepared childbirth". The classes cover two main areas.

Education Approximately 70% of mothers, both primiparae and multiparae, fear labour. Major sources of anxiety include their ability to bear the pain, loss of control over body and emotions,[3] the possibility of medical complications, the baby's health,[4] being restricted to the bed[5] and being in unfamiliar surroundings. A discussion about the processes of pregnancy, labour, and delivery reduces fear of the unknown and serves to dispel a few preconceived ideas. Familiarity with the environment may also help and to this end a tour of the delivery suite is often incorporated into the programme. A discussion on obstetric management, including the possibility of operative delivery, prepares the woman for such an eventuality. A birth plan allows the mother to feel she has some control over her labour and delivery. Most education classes today include a discussion on pain itself. Women are told openly that labour is often painful. A discussion about the nature and severity of the pain and the different pharmacological and non-pharmacological methods of pain relief help women to approach labour with realistic expectations.

Physiotherapy techniques In 1988 Fridh *et al*[6] showed that primiparous, young, emotionally unstable women with unrealistic expectations of

19

childbirth who were the least relaxed suffered the most pain. It is clearly appropriate for women in labour to be as relaxed as possible. Many prepared childbirth classes teach "active relaxation" of mind and body in the belief that tension may impede descent of the presenting part, delay labour and make it more painful. The woman deliberately and systematically relaxes individual muscle groups throughout the body. Some 20% of women can relax naturally and a further 50–60% can be taught to do so. The more practice a woman puts in before labour the easier it is to relax, to relax faster and more profoundly and therefore the more efficacious relaxation becomes in relieving pain. Breathing patterns are also taught at all antenatal classes and a particular emphasis is placed on them by the National Childbirth Trust. The mother is taught how to adapt her breathing to the different stages of labour in order to raise the pain threshold, to maintain relaxation during the stress of labour and to help her cope with the pain. Some classes still teach physical exercises to improve body tone, although this is less common than in the past since there is no evidence that fit, athletic women have easier labours than others.

Antenatal preparation adhering more closely to the teachings of Read and Lamaze is currently experiencing a vogue. It is confusing that the term "Natural Childbirth" previously used to describe Read's methods is today used to describe the situation in which the pregnant woman, with the support of her partner, wishes to maintain control over her labour and delivery, or even simply to describe normal delivery. Learned coping techniques are employed and medical intervention is intended to be kept to an absolute minimum. It covers a spectrum ranging from unmedicated, spontaneous home delivery to hospital delivery. The National Childbirth Trust and the Active Childbirth Movement run private classes that adhere closely to the teachings of Read and Lamaze. The emphasis in these classes is placed on non-pharmacological methods of pain relief and methods of coping with the pain such as breathing control and relaxation exercises. Often there is little or no mention of the intensity of pain likely to be encountered or of pharmacological methods of analgesia, or the possible need for obstetric intervention.

Mechanism of action

Melzack et al[7] described pain as "a complex perceptual experience that is profoundly influenced by psychological variables, such as fear, attention and suggestion", so theoretically clinical pain should be less when anxiety, tension, and fear are reduced. However, the hypothesis that knowledge diminishes fear and so increases resistance to pain is clearly not the whole story, since midwives and female doctors are not immune to painful delivery. Breathing exercises such as the panting taught by Lamaze have an analgesic effect through distraction, similar to the analgesia experienced by a soldier in battle. The mechanism by which antenatal preparation may result in physical advantages may be related to stress hormones. Catecholamines reduce uterine contractility[8,9] and women who are anxious about labour have increased concentrations of plasma catecholamines, longer labours and more birth complications.[8,10–13] Increased anxiety and catecholamine levels in animals have resulted in reduced uterine and placental flow and fetal distress,[14–17] and following the use of sedation or pain relief the fetal condition improved.[17] Measures of maternal anxiety and catecholamine concentrations during labour in humans have also been negatively correlated with fetal well-being, as indicated by cardiotocography.[10]

Efficacy

Read was criticised by physicians of his time because he failed to produce any evidence on the efficacy of his practice. The popularity of antenatal training today suggests that participants derive psychological benefits from it. However, its effect on pain and physical variables remains unresolved. In some studies, women receiving special antenatal training for childbirth have had analgesic requirements similar to those of control women,[18–20] but in most their requirements for pharmacological analgesia are less.[21–26] This does not necessarily imply that these women had less pain, but rather that they were able to tolerate labour and delivery with less analgesia. Melzack et al[7,27] demonstrated a reduction in pain scores after training but the difference was not dramatic and pain scores were still very high even though these women were a self-selected sample with positive attitudes. The average pain reduction depended on the trainer and ranged from 0 to 30%. Even though the best trainer, who taught the orthodox Lamaze technique, achieved pain scores 30% lower than those in unprepared women, more than 80% of trained women had epidural analgesia despite the trainer advising against it. In a group of randomised volunteers, Stevens and Heide[28] demonstrated that prepared childbirth techniques involving relaxation and distraction reduced the pain experience, that is, they produced a true psychological analgesia. Other studies demonstrated little or no effect on pain intensity,[29–31] but found that antenatal training produced a more satisfactory reaction pattern to pain.[30,31]

The physical benefits of antenatal preparation are equally variable. Labours have been claimed to be shorter[26,32–36] or unchanged in length.[18–25,31,37] More spontaneous deliveries with fewer forceps deliveries,[19,21,22,26,38] and a reduced[18,22,25,33,34] or equal incidence[20,23,37] of operative delivery have all been reported. So too have reduced[25,33] or equal blood loss[37] and a lower incidence[18,26] or equal incidence of perineal trauma.[25,37] Reported benefits to the baby include a reduction in fetal distress,[18] less neonatal depression,[33,38] better Apgar scores[39] or equal Apgar scores,[18,21,23] and lower rates of perinatal morbidity and mortality[32,34] and premature labour.[18,19]

Psychological benefits have also been attributed to good antenatal preparation. Fear, anxiety, and apprehension may be less[20] or unchanged.[23,24] The ability to relax,[25,31] to cope with the pain[21] and to maintain self-control[23,30] have been shown to be improved. A lower incidence of postpartum depression,[23,39] greater maternal satisfaction,[23,33,38] a better feeling about the experience for mother and partner,[39] better infant–parent bonding and a more positive attitude to subsequent pregnancies[23] have also been described.

Despite the many positive benefits claimed for psychological preparation these studies should be interpreted with caution since many suffer from methodological shortcomings. A review by Beck and Hall[40] criticises many of the studies for having small numbers,[21,24,36] poor control populations,[19,21,22,24,26] or no controls at all.[32,33,35,38] Many are unblinded and unrandomised[20–22,24,26,36,38,39] and frequently statistical analysis is either inappropriate or completely omitted.[26,32,33,38] Most reports fail to detail variables such as maternal age, fetal weight, oxytocin use, and induction, which influence labour and delivery. Randomisation is particularly important since the type of person selecting prepared childbirth may have a strong influence on outcome. Prepared women tend to be between 20 and 35 years of age,[20] better educated[18,20] with a higher mean family income[20,36] and more positive expectations of childbirth[20] than those who attend no classes. Some[20,24] but not all[23,36] investigations have found pre-treatment anxiety levels to be lower in women seeking antenatal preparation. It is meaningless to compare the labours of two disparate groups and then attribute all the differences to the antenatal preparation. To attempt to overcome this problem Hughey et al[18] compared 500 consecutive Lamaze method deliveries to 500 control patients matched for age, race, parity, and level of education. While use of systemic opioids, duration of labour, oxytocin use, perinatal mortality and postpartum haemorrhage were similar in the two groups, women who had received Lamaze preparation had more spontaneous deliveries, a lower incidence of caesarean section, fetal distress, perineal trauma, and pre-eclampsia. It must be stressed, however, that this was not a randomised study.

There may be several reasons for the variable efficacy of preparation on pain intensity. One explanation may be the severity of labour pain itself. In one survey Melzak[41] found that labour pain for primiparous women without prepared childbirth training was similar to that of amputation of a digit, and in others 60–80% of parturients described labour pain as severe or intolerable.[29,42,43] However, women report a huge variation in pain intensity,[41] ranging from extremely severe to almost none, irrespective of childbirth preparation. Both physical and psychological factors play a part in the perception of pain, a fact that is often neglected during natural childbirth training. Pain scores have been found to correlate positively with frequency of contractions, use of oxytotics, cervical dilatation, the woman's weight, size of the baby, occipito-posterior position, and menstrual pain, as well as anxiety. Maternal age, education, socio-economic status, and emotional support correlate negatively with pain intensity.[7,27,44]

Satisfaction with childbirth is not always closely related to the efficacy of analgesia,[43,45] and this may explain why natural childbirth and psychoprophylaxis remain popular with some women. In the National Birthday Trust survey,[5] approximately 90% of women using relaxation and massage described them as good or very good, although many needed pharmacological analgesia as well. As with other non-pharmacological methods they seem to be good ways of coping with pain, even if they have little or no effect on its severity. In a review by Morgan et al,[45] patients who refused all analgesia had the highest degree of pain but reported high indices of satisfaction. An unsatisfactory maternal experience of childbirth was associated most clearly with forceps delivery and longer labour but not with pain, and the shorter and more natural the labour the greater the proportion satisfied. Similarly, Ranta et al[43] showed a relation between dissatisfaction and instrumental delivery but not with the use of pain relief. Although Paech[46] also found a significant association between instrumental delivery and dissatisfaction with childbirth, he also demonstrated greater satisfaction in women with the lowest pain scores, that is, those who received epidurals, compared with women who received other pharmacological and non-pharmacological methods of pain relief. Furthermore, 5% of women were dissatisfied with the experience of childbirth and the main reason given was inadequate pain relief rather than obstetric factors.

Complications and disadvantages

Although antenatal training techniques may help women to cope with pain, most women still experience severe labour pain.[7,27,29] There is some evidence to suggest that stress-mediated responses may be harmful to both mother and fetus.[8-10,14-16] The often extreme pain of labour is associated with increases in plasma catecholamine concentrations, heart rate, and blood pressure and may cause a reduction in uterine blood flow and fetal asphyxia. These effects may be harmful to a woman with cardiovascular disease and to a fetus with an already reduced oxygen supply. Effective epidural analgesia not only reverses these pain-induced changes but, because of the associated sympathetic blockade, increases uterine blood flow, particularly in pre-eclampsia and other conditions where placental perfusion is compromised.[47-49] Furthermore, elevated catecholamine concentrations may also lead to reduced uterine activity and longer labours.[8] In these circumstances effective epidural analgesia may well be preferable to using psychoprophylaxis alone.

Techniques relying heavily on breathing exercises may lead to hyperventilation with subsequent maternal alkalosis, which impairs placental oxygen transfer, and to vasoconstriction and a reduction in cerebral and uterine blood flow.[50] Similarly, excessive panting may lead to periods of maternal hypoventilation with the possibility of fetal acidosis.

Psychological analgesia places increased demands on the staff. Far more effort and time are required to provide continuous psychological support to women in labour than to give an injection.

Psychological disadvantages have been reported. If natural methods of relieving or coping with pain are over-emphasised many well-intentioned women will think that psychological analgesia is all they will need for a painless labour and delivery. They mistrust caregivers who recommend pharmacological analgesia, but in the event most women who plan not to use medication are unable to carry through this intention[7,51] and feel guilty and a failure. Disparity between maternal expectations and labour experience results in more pain and greater maternal dissatisfaction.[52] Women attending private classes are more likely to be optimistic about non-pharmacological methods of analgesia such as relaxation, breathing exercises, massage, and TENS than those attending NHS classes.[51] It is important to maintain a balanced approach. Rather than to promise a painless labour it is better to suggest that pain is likely to be present, that physical factors may override feelings of psychological "preparedness" and that other methods of pain relief including regional techniques may be necessary. Stewart[53] reported cases of men and women who sought psychotherapy following attempted natural childbirth that had not proceeded as planned. Symptoms of depression, anxiety, and obsessive–compulsive disorders were observed. The women experienced feelings of having "let the side down", of having failed as a woman, of inferiority at being unable to tolerate the pain, and of guilt about "resorting" to an epidural. The male partners felt compelled to stay in the delivery room against their will. Some felt nauseated at the sight of blood or of a partner in such pain, and felt unable to coach and support her. Profound guilt and feelings of failure ensued.

Some purists insist that every delivery should be spontaneous. In the desire to avoid operative delivery the second stage may be unduly prolonged. This may be accompanied by maternal exhaustion, maternal and fetal acidosis, and neonatal depression as well as disappointment for the mother should operative delivery be required. Prepared childbirth training and pharmacological methods of pain relief should be regarded as complementary and compatible procedures rather than mutually exclusive.

Summary

Most couples benefit from antenatal training and its use should be encouraged. However, it should be explained that a woman cannot *choose* to have a normal uncomplicated labour. Many methods of approaching childbirth do not take account of this. The high proportion of women needing conventional analgesia further emphasises the need for a balanced approach. Educational programmes should be designed to give expectant mothers realistic knowledge about what actually happens during labour, the pros and cons of obstetric interventions, obstetric analgesia, and psychological techniques. These programmes, called *prepared* childbirth rather than *natural* childbirth, are to be encouraged. The possibility that a woman may need pharmacological analgesia, including epidural, or obstetric intervention such as episiotomy, forceps or even caesarean section, should be presented in a positive light. Women will then present with realistic expectations and be more relaxed, and the risks of disappointment and feelings of guilt and failure are diminished. Only if the partner really wants to should he be encouraged to attend the delivery. To go through labour using psychological analgesia alone requires strong motivation. It is probably better to encourage an attitude of flexibility during prenatal training rather than a commitment to a prescribed method of coping with labour and delivery.

Support during labour

A friendly atmosphere in the labour ward is a first priority to help a woman cope with pain, and homely surroundings help to allay anxiety and may reduce the need for pharmacological analgesia.[54] Support in labour is an essential part of care and is provided by the attending midwife and, in some cases, a partner or a supportive companion previously unknown to the mother, a "doula".

Midwife   The midwife plays an important role in providing psychological support and encouragement to the parturient. A good midwife with good communication skills goes a long way to allaying fear in labour and may reduce the need for analgesia.[55] Morgan *et al*[56] found that 61% of mothers felt that having a sympathetic midwife to help them through labour was more important than all clinical treatment for pain relief. Furthermore, explanations and participation in decision-making are extremely important factors contributing to maternal relaxation and satisfaction.

Partner   It has long been believed that the presence of the baby's father, or a friend or relative throughout labour to support and encourage the woman helps her to relax and to feel in control and confident. Most women in the USA and the UK have their partners with them during labour and delivery. Active participation by the partner is encouraged to provide psychological support and distraction as well as practical support such as back-rubbing.

Doula The term doula has been used to describe anyone who provides continuous labour support, preferably through to delivery, to soothe, touch, encourage, and explain procedures. A doula is often a lay person, unknown to the parturient before labour, and is more commonly used in societies where it is not normal for the partner to be present during labour and delivery.

Efficacy

Currently there is mounting evidence that continuous intrapartum support, social or professional, in addition to usual hospital care, benefits outcome for both mother and baby. A Cochrane database review[57] of 11 randomised controlled studies[58-68] assessed the effects of continuous intrapartum support on mother and baby compared with the usual hospital care. The studies were extremely diverse. The doula might be an unfamiliar professional (a nurse or midwife), a paid or voluntary lay person, or a chosen, familiar support person. The countries of origin were equally diverse: Europe, Canada, South America, South Africa and the USA. Hospital obstetric routines and conditions differed, ranging from the less medically developed Guatemala in the early 1980s[59] to a modern hospital in the USA in the 1990s where significantly more control is exerted over the progress of labour.[60] Equally diverse were the obstetric risk status of the women and whether or not a husband, partner or significant other person known to the mother was also allowed to be present. In all studies the support person was there to encourage, touch, reassure, and praise the mother and to provide positive support and companionship.

Despite these large differences in study design the outcomes were remarkably similar. Whether or not a familiar companion was also allowed, the continuous presence of a trained support person who was unknown to the woman before labour, improved both physiological and psychological aspects of labour, delivery, and the postpartum period. There was a reduction in duration of labour, oxytocin use and operative vaginal delivery rate. Neonatal outcome was also improved. The incidence of 5-minute Apgar scores of less than 7 was reduced and fewer babies required transfer to the neonatal intensive care unit or prolonged hospitalisation for longer than 48 hours after delivery. Analgesic requirements were also reduced. Kennell *et al*[60] showed that epidural analgesia was required seven times more frequently in controls than in the supported group, although the use of systemic opioids was not significantly different. Hofmeyr *et al*[58] showed no difference in the number of women requesting pethidine analgesia, although supported women required the first dose later in labour and there was a trend towards an increased use of multiple doses in the control group. The need for caesarean section was also reduced by the presence of a trained support person, in studies where support from a significant other person was not allowed. Four trials found supported mothers to be less likely to score the childbirth experience negatively. Anxiety scores were reduced, the overall experience of childbirth and sense of being in control during childbirth were scored more highly, and there were fewer reports of feeling tense during labour and finding labour worse than expected.

Why might the presence of a doula, either lay person or midwife, have such positive effect, if indeed it does? Maternal anxiety has been linked with disturbances in labour progress and fetal well-being[8,10,13] for reasons already described. A doula may have an important role in reducing anxiety and therefore catecholamine concentrations, and in so doing, facilitate uterine contractility and utero-placental blood flow. Pain perception is influenced by psychological variables including anxiety[7] and this may explain why the presence of a doula resulted in a reduction in analgesic requirements in some studies.

Since many of the positive results attributed to the presence of a doula occurred whether or not a partner, friend or relative was present, it appears that the support of a chosen person is no substitute for the support provided by a specially trained caregiver. The reasons for this are not clear but it may be related to the amount of "hands-on" support provided by a doula. Bertsch *et al*[69] showed better results when a female companion (doula) was present rather than a first-time father. During periods of maternal discomfort the doula touched the mother in some way 95% of the time whereas male partners did so less than 20% of the time. Males were also present for less time and were close to the mother less often. A partner has a personal involvement with the woman and lacks the experience of labour, and so may not have the same positive impact. A doula may engender greater feelings of confidence. The fact that a caregiver is previously unknown to the mother may help the mother to avoid feelings of having to meet expectations or keep up appearances which may occur when supported by a friend or family member.

Implications

The presence of continuous intrapartum support is perhaps of even greater importance in these days of modern obstetric practices than in the past. Over the past 40 years there has been an increased use of new technology in labour, creating a more clinical environment which may undermine the woman's

27

confidence, self-esteem and sense of control. In most centres the role of doula falls solely on the midwife, yet with the increase in workload she has less time to support a woman in labour, in particular the amount of "hands-on" care she can give is less. Other tasks include starting infusions, monitoring vital signs, attaching and adjusting monitors, writing notes, performing vaginal examinations, and monitoring the progress of labour, all of which limit the support that the midwife can provide. Within the financial constraints of the NHS, staff shortages are common and a midwife is not infrequently required to care for more than one labouring woman at a time. This issue needs to be addressed, not only because of the obvious benefit to the mother and baby of experienced lay support, but because of the financial benefit too. Flexible staffing of the labour ward to match the number of midwives to the number of women in labour would help. Otherwise provision of a specially trained support person should be considered as an adjunct to conventional analgesia and routine obstetric and midwifery care.

Hypnosis

Hypnosis is the oldest form of psychological analgesia dating back for thousands of years. It is used in several NHS pain clinics to treat the pain of shingles, back injury, arthritis and cancer. A few units in the UK provide it for pain relief and amnesia during labour and delivery, but compared with more conventional forms of analgesia its use is not widespread. Hypnosis, acupuncture, and homeopathy together are used by fewer than 0·5% of women[51] for labour and delivery.

Suggestion forms the basis of hypnotherapy. A hypnotised subject appears to be asleep, often with eyes closed, and very relaxed. In reality the patient is awake but in a trance, a state of deep concentration in which the subject is very receptive to suggestion, and near absolute credence is given to the suggestions of the hypnotist. Pleasurable sensations are suggested and distressing inputs such as abdominal pain are transformed to more tolerable thoughts such as "tightenings" or "waves rolling in from the sea"[70] while perineal pain becomes "pressure". Pain can be better controlled than in the normal wide-awake state.

Success with this method as a means of pain relief in labour requires a great deal of antenatal training. The woman has to attend several conditioning or training classes, run by a skilled hypnotist, in order to reach the degree of concentration required for labour. During the classes a trance is induced, often by the eye fixation technique to produce retinal fatigue, or by the instructor's repeating words and phrases in a monotonous, soft hypnotic voice, producing progressive relaxation by voice suggestion. Positive suggestions are then given of the diminished awareness of pain, diminished need for pharmacological analgesia, and the ability to produce anaesthesia of the perineum for the delivery of the baby's head. The satisfaction and pleasure of childbirth is often stressed. The woman is taught slow rhythmic breathing throughout. The woman is then awakened with suggestions of wakening and feeling refreshed. Best results during labour are achieved if the woman is hypnotised professionally. However, to have the hypnotist present for most of the labour may be prohibitively expensive. Alternatively a woman may use self-hypnosis but the success rate is less. Brann and Guzvica[70] used an audio-cassette of an 'in labour' programme with instructions to enter a hypnotised state and the sound of the sea in the background, so avoiding the need for the hypnotist to be present.

The labour ward staff need to know how to care for a hypnotised woman during labour. Anything which may affect her ability to concentrate should be avoided, with noise kept to a minimum. Whilst systemic opioids may interfere with the ability to concentrate, it is claimed that they frequently heighten the hypnotic effect.[71] The application of hypnosis is limited. Only about 25% of women can be hypnotised to a depth at which the appreciation of pain is substantially reduced.[72-75] Some women are partly susceptible and 10–20% are not susceptible at all.[76,77] The eye-roll test[78] grades the ability to roll the eyes upwards and is a commonly used test of susceptibility to hypnosis.

Efficacy

Hypnosis has been claimed to reduce pain and the requirement for pharmacological analgesia,[70,71,75,77,79,80] and to shorten labour.[70,71,75,79,80] Efficacy is difficult to assess since there are few trials published, few are randomised[81] and some even have no controls.[82,83] Using self-hypnosis in volunteer parturients, Davidson[79] showed that 53% of women experienced minimal or no pain during labour and delivery compared with 6% in the control group, and 59% of women required no other analgesia compared with 2% of controls. Similarly Gross and Posner[71] found volunteer hypnotised primips were four times less likely to require conventional analgesia than controls. However, frequently analgesia is considered inadequate even in women regarded as suitable hypnotic subjects. Three further unrandomised studies demonstrated 60–78% of women required additional analgesia.[70,83,84] Success is greater in multips than in primips[71,83] and for spontaneous rather than instrumental delivery.[71] In the only randomised controlled trial of hypnosis in labour, Freeman et al[81] found no difference in epidural use between the two groups, but good or moderate hypnotic subjects were less likely to require epidural analgesia than poor hypnotic subjects. Scores for pain relief were similar between the two groups, and between good and poor hypnotic subjects.

29

The differences in susceptibility to hypnosis as well as in the physical perception of pain may, in part, explain why the effect of hypnosis is so variable, ranging from none, through "taking the edge off", to providing a virtually pain-free labour. In a really deep trance, analgesia so complete as to allow a caesarean section or hysterectomy without any other analgesia or anaesthesia has been reported.[71]

Effect on labour

In unrandomised reviews, Davidson[79] and Gross and Posner[71] reported a reduction in the duration of the first stage of labour by nearly 50% among hypnotised subjects, confirming earlier findings from the 1950s.[75,80] However, this was not supported by the later study of Winkelstein in 1958,[77] while in a randomised study Freeman et al[81] found labour was significantly *prolonged* in the hypnotised group.

Whether or not hypnosis provides effective pain relief it appears to make labour more satisfying and a more pleasant experience for many of those who are susceptible.[70,79,81]

Mechanism of action

It is well known that psychological factors affect the perception of pain[85] and the state of altered consciousness produced by hypnosis takes this to the extreme. Although the exact mode of action is uncertain, the hypnotised subject is able to prevent unpleasant inputs, including pain, from reaching consciousness.

Effects on the baby

There are no known detrimental effects on the baby and some reports suggest a reduction in perinatal morbidity. Moya and James[84] demonstrated, not surprisingly, that babies born to hypnotised mothers were more alert, had better Apgar scores and more effective respiration than those whose mothers received cyclopropane anaesthesia. If mothers received regional analgesia there was no difference, suggesting the advantage of hypnosis was only in the avoidance of depressant drugs. Furthermore, no such beneficial effects have been demonstrated since.[70,71]

Disadvantages and complications

Hypnosis involves much antenatal training which is time-consuming and may be expensive. Through amnesia the woman may feel deprived of the sense of active participation in the birth. Suggestion to the mother to breathe deeply may result in hyperventilation tetany[84] and maternal alkalosis may reduce fetal oxygenation[86] (see Chapter 4, Nitrous oxide). It has been suggested that hypnosis may lead to psychological problems later on,[73,74] manifest either as subtle changes or overt psychotic or anxiety states, particularly in women who wish totally to avoid any experience of labour and delivery.[73] Hypnosis should therefore be avoided in any woman with psychotic or neurotic tendencies.

Summary

It would be difficult to recommend hypnosis for routine use in labour and delivery in view of its unpredictable efficacy and the large proportion of women who require additional analgesia. However, hypnosis does appear to help a subset of women and a trial of hypnosis in labour should not be denied.

Biofeedback

Biofeedback is on the borderline between psychological and physical methods of analgesia. Relaxation is a major component of psychological preparation for childbirth and is claimed to relieve pain, reduce anxiety, and speed labour. Biofeedback techniques are used outside the obstetric field as a method of relaxation training to reduce stress, and they can be taught to, and practised by, parturients during the antenatal period for use in labour. Two methods have been described. Electromyographic (muscular) relaxation involves the voluntary relaxation of muscles while muscle tension, measured by electromyography, is fed back to the patient in the form of audible clicks through an earpiece. Successful voluntary-muscle relaxation is indicated by a reduced click frequency. The skin-conductance method uses sweating as a measure of sympathetic activity and therefore of stress. Relaxation results in a reduced skin conductance heard as a decreased rate of clicks. During training parturients are taught relaxation techniques. A cut-off threshold is set on the biofeedback apparatus and if a desired level of relaxation is reached the clicks cease. A more sensitive threshold can be used as training progresses.

Few trials have been conducted on biofeedback in labour and these have been small, with large possibilities for bias. In a small randomised trial using untreated controls Duchene[87] claimed to have demonstrated reduced pain scores in the biofeedback group but no data were given in the published results to support that claim. A randomised study by St James-Roberts *et al*[88] compared women taught electromyographic and skin-conductance biofeedback techniques with controls receiving the usual antenatal relaxation and education classes. No significant differences were found in duration of labour, use of pharmacological analgesia, instrumental delivery rate and neonatal welfare. A review of studies by the Cochrane database[89]

31

was inconclusive. It stated that biofeedback may or may not be a useful form of non-pharmacological pain relief in labour and may or may not have a beneficial effect on the operative delivery rate but the current studies did not help to solve these issues. In view of these findings and the requirements for equipment, time, practice, and a very motivated mother, biofeedback techniques are rarely employed in labour.

References

1 Read GD. *Natural childbirth.* London: Heinemann, 1933.
2 Lamaze F. *Painless childbirth: psychoprophylatic method* (Celestin CB, translator). London: Burke Publishing Company, 1958.
3 Lederman R. *Psychosocial adaptation in pregnancy.* Englewood Cliffs, NJ: Prentice-Hall, 1984.
4 Read GD. *Childbirth without fear.* New York: Harper Brothers, 1944.
5 Wraight A. Coping with pain. In: Chamberlain G, Wraight A, Steer P, eds. *Pain and its relief in childbirth: the results of a national survey conducted by the National Birthday Trust.* Edinburgh: Churchill Livingstone, 1993:79–92.
6 Fridh G, Kopare T, Gaston-Johansson F, Norvell KT. *Res Nurs Health* 1988;**11**:117–24.
7 Melzack R, Taenzer P, Feldman P, Kinch RA. Labour is still painful after prepared childbirth training. *Can Med Assoc J* 1981;**125**:357–63.
8 Lederman RP, Lederman E, Work BA Jr, McCann DS. The relationship of maternal anxiety, plasma catecholamines, and plasma cortisol to progress in labor. *Am J Obstet Gynecol* 1978;**132**:495–500.
9 Zuspan FP, Cibils LA, Pose SV. Myometrial and cardiovascular responses to alterations in plasma epinephrine and norepinephrine. *Am J Obstet Gynecol* 1962;**84**:841–51.
10 Lederman RP, Lederman E, Work B Jr, McCann DS. Anxiety and epinephrine in multiparous women in labor: relationship to duration of labor and fetal heart rate pattern. *Am J Obstet Gynecol* 1985;**153**:870–7.
11 McDonald RL. Personality characteristics in patients with three obstetric complications. *Psychosom Med* 1965;**27**:383–90.
12 McDonald RL, Gynther MD, Christakos AC. Relations between maternal anxiety and obstetric complications. *Psychosom Med* 1963;**25**:357–63.
13 Davids A, DeVault S. Maternal anxiety during pregnancy and childbirth abnormalities. *Psychosom Med* 1962;**24**:464–70.
14 Adamsons K, Mueller-Heubach E, Myers RE. Production of fetal asphyxia in the rhesus monkey by administration of catecholamines to the mother. *Am J Obstet Gynecol* 1971; **109**:248–62.
15 Myers RE. Maternal psychological stress and fetal asphyxia: a study in the monkey. *Am J Obstet Gynecol* 1975;**122**:47–59.
16 Shnider SM, Wright RG, Levinson G *et al.* Uterine blood flow and plasma norepinephrine changes during maternal stress in the pregnant ewe. *Anesthesiology* 1979;**50**:524–7.
17 Morishima HO, Yeh M-N, James LS. Reduced uterine blood flow and fetal hypoxemia with acute maternal stress: experimental observation in the pregnant baboon. *Am J Obstet Gynecol* 1979;**134**:270–5.
18 Hughey MJ, McElin TW, Young T. Maternal and fetal outcome of Lamaze-prepared patients. *Obstet Gynecol* 1978;**51**:643–7.
19 Rodway HE. Education for childbirth and its results. *J Obstet Gynaecol Br Emp* 1957; **64**:545–60.
20 Davis CD, Morrone FA. An objective evaluation of a prepared childbirth program. *Am J Obstet Gynecol* 1962;**84**:1196–206.
21 Scott JR, Rose NB. Effect of psychoprophylaxis (Lamaze preparation) on labor and delivery in primiparas. *N Engl J Med* 1976;**294**:1205–7.

22 Laird MD, Hogan M. An elective program on preparation for childbirth at the Sloane Hospital for Women, May, 1951, to June, 1953. *Am J Obstet Gynecol* 1956;**72**:641–7.
23 Huttel FA, Mitchell I, Fischer WM, Meyer A-E. A quantitative evaluation of psychoprophylaxis in childbirth. *J Psychosom Res* 1972;**16**:81–92.
24 Zax M, Sameroff AJ, Farnum JE. Childbirth education, maternal attitudes, and delivery. *Am J Obstet Gynecol* 1975;**123**:185–90.
25 Roberts H, Wootton IDP, Kane KM, Harnett WE. The value of antenatal preparation. *J Obstet Gynaecol Br Emp* 1953;**60**:404–8.
26 Van Auken WBD, Tomlinson DR. An appraisal of patient training for childbirth. *Am J Obstet Gynecol* 1953;**66**:100–5.
27 Melzack R, Kinch R, Dobkin P, Lebrun M, Taenzer P. Severity of labour pain: influence of physical as well as psychologic variables. *Can Med Assoc J* 1984;**130**:579–84.
28 Stevens RJ, Heide F. Analgesic characteristics of prepared childbirth techniques: attention focusing and systematic relaxation. *J Psychosom Res* 1977;**21**:429–38.
29 Bundsen P, Peterson L-E, Selstam U. Pain relief during delivery. An evaluation of conventional methods. *Acta Obstet Gynecol Scand* 1982;**61**:289–97.
30 Javert CT, Hardy JD. Measurement of pain intensity in labor and its physiologic, neurologic and pharmacologic implications. *Am J Obstet Gynecol* 1950;**60**:552–63.
31 Davenport-Slack B, Boylan CH. Psychological correlates of childbirth pain. *Psychosom Med* 1974;**36**:215–23.
32 Thoms H, Wyatt RH. One thousand consecutive deliveries under a training for childbirth program. *Am J Obstet Gynecol* 1951;**61**:205–9.
33 Thoms H, Karlovsky ED. Two thousand deliveries under a training for childbirth program. *Am J Obstet Gynecol* 1954;**68**:279–84.
34 Miller HL. Education for childbirth. *Obstet Gynecol* 1961;**17**:120–3.
35 Yahia C, Ulin PR. Preliminary experience with a psychophysical program of preparation for childbirth. *Am J Obstet Gynecol* 1965;**93**:942–9.
36 Leonard RF. Evaluation of selection tendencies of patients preferring prepared childbirth. *Obstet Gynecol* 1973;**42**:371–7.
37 Burnett CWF. The value of antenatal exercises. *J Obstet Gynaecol Br Emp* 1956;**63**: 40–57.
38 Tupper C. Conditioning for childbirth. *Am J Obstet Gynecol* 1956;**71**:733–40.
39 Enkin MW, Smith SL, Dermer SW, Emmett JO. An adequately controlled study of the effectiveness of PPM training. In: Morris N, ed. *Psychosomatic medicine in obstetrics and gynaecology*, Basle: S. Karger, 1972:62–7.
40 Beck NC, Hall D. Natural Childbirth. A review and analysis. *Obstet Gynecol* 1978;**52**: 371–9.
41 Melzack R. The myth of painless childbirth. *Pain* 1984;**19**:321–37.
42 Kangas-Saarela T, Kangas-Kärki K. Pain and pain relief in labour: parturients' experiences. *Int J Obstet Anesth* 1994;**3**:67–74.
43 Ranta P, Spalding M, Kangas-Saarela T *et al.* Maternal expectations and experiences of labour pain-options of 1091 Finnish parturients. *Acta Anaesth Scand* 1995;**39**:60–6.
44 Brown ST, Campbell D, Kurtz A. Characteristics of labor pain at two stages of cervical dilatation. *Pain* 1989;**38**:289–95.
45 Morgan BM, Bulpitt CJ, Clifton P, Lewis PJ. Analgesia and satisfaction in childbirth (The Queen Charlotte's 1000 mother survey). *Lancet* 1982;**ii**:808–10.
46 Paech MJ. The King Edward Memorial Hospital 1000 mother survey of methods of pain relief in labour. *Anaesth Intens Care* 1991;**19**:393–9.
47 Jouppila R, Puolakka J, Kauppila A, Vuori J. Maternal and umbilical cord plasma noradrenaline concentrations during labour with and without segmental extradural analgesia, and during caesarean section. *Br J Anaesth* 1984;**56**:251–5.
48 Abboud T, Artal R, Sarkis F, Henriksen EH, Kammula RK. Sympathoadrenal activity, maternal, fetal, and neonatal responses after epidural anesthesia in the preeclamptic patient. *Am J Obstet Gynecol* 1982;**144**:915–18.
49 Hollmén AI, Jouppila R, Jouppila P, Koivula A, Vierola H. Effect of extradural analgesia using bupivacaine and 2-chloroprocaine on intervillous blood flow during normal labour. *Br J Anaesth* 1982;**54**:837–42.

33

50 Levinson G, Shnider SM, deLorimier AA, Steffenson JL. Effects of maternal hyperventilation on uterine blood flow and fetal oxygenation and acid-base status. *Anesthesiology* 1974;**40**:340–7.

51 Steer P. The methods of pain relief used. In: Chamberlain G, Wraight A, Steer P, eds. *Pain and its relief in childbirth: the results of a national survey conducted by the National Birthday Trust.* Edinburgh: Churchill Livingstone, 1993:49–67.

52 Astbury J. Labour pain: the role of childbirth education, information and expectation. In: Peck C, Wallace M, eds. *Problems in pain.* Oxford: Pergamon Press, 1980:245–51.

53 Stewart DE. Psychiatric symptoms following attempted natural childbirth. *Can Med Assoc J* 1982;**127**:713–16.

54 Chapman MG, Jones M, Spring JE, De Swiet M, Chamberlain GVP. The use of a birthroom: a randomized controlled trial comparing delivery with that in the labour ward. *Br J Obstet Gynaecol* 1986;**93**:182–7.

55 Waldenström U. Midwives' attitudes to pain relief during labour and delivery. *Midwifery* 1988;**4**:48–57.

56 Morgan BM, Bulpitt CJ, Clifton P, Lewis PJ. The consumers' attitude to obstetric care. *Br J Obstet Gynaecol* 1984;**91**:624–8.

57 Keirse MJNC, Enkin M, Lumley J. Support from caregivers during childbirth. In: *The Cochrane Pregnancy and Childbirth Database. The Cochrane Collaboration and Update Software*, 1995, Issue 1.

58 Hofmeyr GJ, Nikodem VC, Wolman W-L, Chalmers BE, Kramer T. Companionship to modify the clinical birth environment: effects on progress and perceptions of labour, and breastfeeding. *Br J Obstet Gynaecol* 1991;**98**:756–64.

59 Sosa R, Kennell J, Klaus M, Robertson S, Urrutia J. The effect of a supportive companion on perinatal problems, length of labor and mother-infant interaction. *N Engl J Med* 1980;**303**:597–600.

60 Kennell J, Klaus M, McGrath S, Robertson S, Hinkley C. Continuous emotional support during labor in a US hospital. A randomized controlled trial. *JAMA* 1991;**265**:2197–201.

61 Klaus MH, Kennell JH, Robertson SS, Sosa R. Effects of social support during parturition on maternal and infant morbidity. *BMJ* 1986;**293**:585–7.

62 Wolman W-L, Chalmers B, Hofmeyr J, Nikodem VC. Postpartum depression and companionship in the clinical birth environment: a randomized, controlled study. *Am J Obstet Gynecol* 1993;**168**:1388–93.

63 Hodnett ED, Osborn RW. A randomized trial of the effects of monitrice support during labor: mothers' views two to four weeks postpartum. *Birth* 1989;**16**:177–83.

64 Bréart G, Garel M, Mlika-Cabane N. Evaluation of different policies of management of labour for primiparous women. Trial B: results of the continuous professional support trial. *Evaluation in pre-, peri-, and post-natal care delivery systems* 1992:57–68.

65 Bréart G, Mlika-Cabane N, Kaminski M *et al.* Evaluation of different policies for the management of labour. *Early Hum Dev* 1992;**29**:309–12.

66 Cogan R, Spinnato JA. Social support during premature labor: effects on labor and the newborn. *J Psychosom Obstet Gynaecol* 1988;**8**:209–16.

67 Hemminki E, Virta A-L, Koponen P, Malin M, Kojo-Austin H, Tuimala R. A trial on continuous human support during labor: feasibility, interventions and mothers' satisfaction. *J Psychosom Obstet Gynaecol* 1990;**11**:239–50.

68 Hodnett ED, Osborn RW. Effects of continuous intrapartum professional support on childbirth outcomes. *Res Nurs Hlth* 1989;**12**:289–97.

69 Bertsch TD. Labor support by first-time fathers: direct observations with a comparison to experienced doulas. *J Psychosom Obstet Gynaecol* 1990;**11**:251–60.

70 Brann LR, Guzvica SA. Comparison of hypnosis with conventional relaxation for antenatal and intrapartum use: a feasibility study in general practice. *J R Coll Gen Pract* 1987;**37**:437–40.

71 Gross HN, Posner NA. An evaluation of hypnosis for obstetric delivery. *Am J Obstet Gynecol* 1963;**87**:912–20.

72 Steer P. The availability of pain relief. In: Chamberlain G, Wraight A, Steer P, eds. *Pain and its relief in childbirth: the results of a national survey conducted by the National Birthday Trust.* Edinburgh: Churchill Livingstone, 1993:45–8.

73 Wahl CW. Contraindications and limitations of hypnosis in obstetric analgesia. *Am J Obstet Gynecol* 1962;**84**:1869–72.

74 Rosen H. Hypnosis-applications and misapplications. *JAMA* 1960;**172**:683–7.

75 Abramson M, Heron WT. An objective evaluation of hypnosis in obstetrics. Preliminary report. *Am J Obstet Gynecol* 1950;**59**:1069–74.

76 Plantevin OM. *Analgesia and anaesthesia in obstetrics*. London: Butterworths, 1973:19.

77 Winkelstein LB. Routine hypnosis for obstetrical delivery. An evaluation of hypnosuggestion in 200 consecutive cases. *Am J Obstet Gynecol* 1958;**76**:152–60.

78 Spiegel H, Spiegel D. *Trance and treatment*. New York: Basic Books, 1978:1–77.

79 Davidson JA. An assessment of the value of hypnosis in pregnancy and labour. *BMJ* 1962;**ii**:951–3.

80 Michael AM. Hypnosis in childbirth. *BMJ* 1952;**i**:734–7.

81 Freeman RM, Macaulay AJ, Eve L, Chamberlain GVP, Bhat AV. Randomised trial of self hypnosis for analgesia in labour. *BMJ* 1986;**292**:657–8.

82 Fry A. Hypnosis as an anaesthetic and analgesic in midwifery. *The Practitioner* 1959;**183**:338–42.

83 Tom KS. Hypnosis in obstetrics and gynecology. *Obstet Gynecol* 1960;**16**:222–6.

84 Moya F, James LS. Medical hypnosis for obstetrics. *JAMA* 1960;**174**:2026–32.

85 Melzack R, Wall PD. Pain mechanisms: a new theory. *Science* 1965;**150**:971–9.

86 Motoyama EK, Rivard G, Acheson F, Cook CD. Adverse effect of maternal hyperventilation on the foetus. *Lancet* 1966;**i**:286–8.

87 Duchene P. Effects of biofeedback on childbirth pain. *J Pain Sympt Manage* 1989;**4**:117–23.

88 St James-Roberts I, Hutchinson C, Haran F, Chamberlain G. Biofeedback as an aid to childbirth. *Br J Obstet Gynaecol* 1983;**90**:56–60.

89 Simkin P. Biofeedback in prenatal class attenders. In: *The Cochrane pregnancy and childbirth database*. The Cochrane collaboration and update software, 1995, Issue 1.

3: Physical methods of pain relief

Transcutaneous electrical nerve stimulation (TENS)

Massage

Acupuncture

Water baths

Water blocks

Intradermal "anaesthesia"

Abdominal decompression

Aromatherapy

Audioanalgesia

Homeopathy

Herbalism

Transcutaneous electrical nerve stimulation (TENS)

Transcutaneous electrical nerve stimulation has been used for the relief of chronic pain since the 1970s and was introduced for use in childbirth in the early 1980s. Although TENS is often referred to as an important component of labour analgesia, it is not used extensively. In the 1990 National Birthday Trust survey[1] it was used by only 5% of women and mainly during the early stages of labour. Its use was, however, more widespread than that of other non-pharmacological methods of analgesia.

Two pairs of electrodes are adhered to the back on each side of the vertebral column, over the posterior primary rami of T10–L1 and S2–4 (Figure 3.1). Wires connect them to a small battery-powered pulse generator which produces electrical pulses of 0·1–0·5 ms duration, at a frequency of 0–200 Hz depending on the model used although for labour 40–150 Hz is used. The current is gradually increased by the woman until a tingling sensation is felt. The maximum tolerated amplitude is used whilst maintaining a pleasant sensation and the amplitude can be increased up to a maximum of 50 mA as labour progresses. This background stimulation is used between the contractions. During a contraction the stimulation can be increased[2] and then returned to background level after the contraction

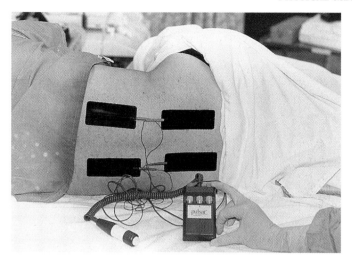

FIGURE 3.1—*Position of TENS electrodes*

has subsided. Usually 5–10 mA is used as background stimulation and 25–40 mA for the boost during a contraction.

TENS appears to work best for low level pain and is therefore at its most effective earlier on in labour.[3] It is most efficacious for back pain[2,4–6] but has little effect on abdominal or suprapubic pain[5–7] or perineal pain.[4,8] Hence, pain relief during the second stage is negligible.[2,3,5,8,9] The additional pain felt during the second stage is mainly due to stretch and tearing of perineal structures innervated by somatic nerves, comprising mainly A fibres, and these impulses are not reduced by further stimulation with TENS. Furthermore, many women switch it off during the second stage because it distracts them from breathing and pushing.[8] Some authors have suggested placing the electrodes over the area of pain even if this does not correspond to the dermatomal levels of the uterus and cervix.[5,6] This method appears to work for low back pain,[6] but whilst Robson claimed "great relief" in two patients by placing electrodes suprapubically,[2] later work has failed to confirm this success.[6]

Mechanisms of action

Mechanism of pain transmission

Pain impulses are transmitted via visceral nerves along slow conducting Aδ and C fibres which enter the spinal cord through nerve roots T10–L1. Pain is referred to the areas (dermatomes) supplied by the same nerve roots, that is, the lower abdomen. Uterine contractions are often also felt in the lower back because pain inputs from the uterus entering the spinal cord

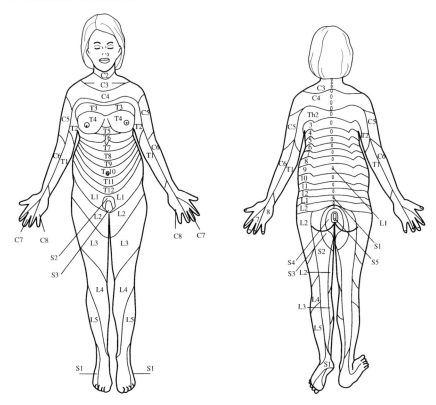

FIGURE 3.2—*Dermatomes: for areas of relevance to pain in labour, see text*

through the anterior primary rami of T10–L1 are felt as referred pain over the area supplied by the posterior rami, the skin overlying the L2–S2 vertebrae (Figure 3.2). Some women experience continuous low back pain and some feel contraction pains primarily in the back.[10] Continuous low back pain in labour is often associated with an occipito-posterior position, stretching in particular the posterior part of the lower segment of the uterus, the cervix and other pain-sensitive structures in the pelvis. Additional pain during the transitional stage and second stage of labour is caused by distension of the vagina and perineum and from pressure on and stretching of adjacent structures. Some of these pain impulses are transmitted through visceral nerves but the main route is via somatic afferents of the sacral plexus, entering the cord through the pudendal nerves and the S2–4 nerve roots. Pain is both localised to the site of pain activation and referred, and is felt in the perineal, perianal, sacral and suprapubic areas.

Aδ and C pain fibres enter the spinal cord through the dorsal nerve roots and synapse mainly in the substantia gelatinosa, lamina II, of the dorsal

38

horn. They communicate with neurones with cell bodies in lamina V that ascend to the brain and the neurotransmitter at this synapse is largely substance P. Transmission can be inhibited by fibres descending in the dorsolateral funiculus from the brain stem and by collaterals from sensory neurones in the same spinal segment carrying myelinated Aβ fibres which ascend in the dorsal columns. Most inhibitory inputs act through interneurones causing presynaptic inhibition of the pain transmission.

Mechanism of action of TENS

TENS is thought to relieve labour pain in two ways. High frequency TENS most commonly used in labour may act by stimulating the myelinated Aβ fibres in the posterior primary rami of the spinal nerve roots T10–L1 and S2–4, the collaterals of which synapse in the substantia gelatinosa, activating neurones that inhibit transmitter release along pain pathways. Cortical impulses from higher centres can also act via the descending inhibitory neurones, hence the value of mental distraction on the pain threshold.

It has been suggested that continuous use of low frequency stimulation at 2 Hz acts through neuronal release of endorphins and that the release of endorphins into the cerebrospinal fluid (CSF) may result in a feeling of well-being as well as analgesia. This theory is based on direct evidence following examination of the CSF.[11] The partial reversal by naloxone of analgesia produced by low frequency stimulation[12,13] provides indirect evidence of endogenous opioid release, although this has not been reproduced by later investigators. What is more generally accepted is that high frequency or conventional TENS is not affected by naloxone and may exert its action by release of some other humoral product not yet identified.

Efficacy

The effect of TENS on the pain of labour and delivery is equivocal. Early uncontrolled trials suggested it was helpful for 75–90% of women.[2,3,9] In a controlled but unrandomised study, Miller Jones[8] found similar results whereby 72% of women obtained satisfactory pain relief and primiparae in the TENS group required significantly less pethidine than controls. However, in subsequent randomised controlled and blinded trials comparing TENS with dummy TENS, results were far less positive, showing no benefit with TENS in terms of pain relief and the need for other forms of analgesia.[14,15] Only 14% of women were reported to have good pain relief in the study by Nesheim[15] and Harrison et al[14] found only 12% of primips completed labour without additional analgesia. In a large, prospective, randomised, double-blind, placebo-controlled trial by Thomas et al,[7] results were similar. There was no difference in pain intensity between women using TENS and those using dummy TENS, nor was there any difference between the two groups in change of pain experienced when the machine was switched off for two contractions each hour. Furthermore the need for supplementary analgesia was similar in the two groups.

Although some women undoubtedly do achieve pain relief with TENS in early labour, even then it is rarely complete and a large number of women experience no benefit at all, particularly in late labour. Figures quoted range from 12% upwards,[2,3,8,9,16] with Bundsen et al[5] finding nearly 80% of primiparae had severe to almost unbearable pain. In a recent survey of maternal satisfaction,[17] 22% of women using TENS found it helpful but nearly the same number, 20%, found it unhelpful and this was the highest negative score for any method of pain relief. Results were similar to those for pethidine and worse than for nitrous oxide. In the same survey women who were intending to use TENS alone were less likely to succeed than with any other intended form of pain relief, including "no analgesia".

It is difficult to assess the efficacy of TENS for several reasons. It is used early in labour and therefore cannot be compared with methods required later on, women are reluctant to remove the TENS later in labour to assess how bad the pain would be without it and there is a significant placebo effect. One such observation was that 40% of women receiving dummy TENS experienced more pain when the machine was "switched off".[7] Similarly, in another study,[18] although 93% of patients using TENS achieved good to excellent pain relief, this extent of pain relief was also claimed by 62% receiving placebo TENS. Despite the lack of evidence for analgesic efficacy, many women make favourable comments and say they would use it again in a future labour.[3,7,8,14]

Indications and contraindications

TENS is a non-invasive technique which allows the mother to maintain a degree of control over her own pain relief and to remain mobile. It can be used at home and can be applied by a trained midwife. TENS cannot be used in water, with electro-acupuncture or in the presence of a pacemaker, a rare occurrence among women of childbearing age. The siting of the electrodes precludes its use with back massage and with epidural analgesia, although in the latter situation it should not be necessary.

Side effects and complications

TENS is remarkably free of side effects, the most common being a rash which occurs occasionally at the electrode sites.[19] Some women dislike the tingling sensation around the electrode sites, which increases with strength of stimulation.[2,3] Earlier machines produced artefactual recordings of the fetal heart signal when TENS was used simultaneously with internal monitoring.[5] Current TENS machines have a filter to prevent this problem.[20] Furthermore, the low current density of modern TENS machines has been shown not to induce irregularities in the fetal heart,[20] a potential problem with earlier models.

Not all hospitals provide TENS units and a woman led to believe in TENS may feel constrained to provide it for herself. Units can be hired from large chemists. Although she need not pay the £150–£200 cost of buying the unit, she nevertheless incurs a cost when she hires and some women have reported they feel cheated by this.

Effects on labour

A retrospective study by Kubista et al[21] suggested that TENS was associated with a shorter duration of labour, although this study was unrandomised and it is more likely that a shorter labour allows a woman to survive with TENS alone rather than TENS having an effect on labour itself. Randomised controlled studies have shown no effect on labour duration.[6,14]

Effects on the baby

There are no known harmful effects to the baby. In fact, Bundsen et al[5] claimed that infants born to TENS-treated mothers had better Apgar scores than controls. However, this was an unrandomised, retrospective study and this finding has not been reproduced.[8]

Monitoring and management

The technique of using TENS needs to be explained and this is done best before labour, when the woman is not in pain. Hiring a TENS machine before labour enables the mother to practise with it before labour begins. This may help to improve efficacy and it can then be used at home in the early stages of labour when it is most likely to be effective. Not all midwives are trained in the use of TENS. Furthermore, the UKCC has ruled it cannot be approved for use by midwives on their own responsibility. Some units have trained midwives who are then supervised by physiotherapists in its use.

Summary

TENS may provide limited pain relief during the first stage of labour. However, women rarely get through without requiring supplementary analgesia and those that do tend to be those with shorter labours. In order to prevent women from feeling they have been misled and cheated when they experience no benefit, it is important to stress beforehand that TENS alone may not provide sufficient analgesia for the whole of labour. Nevertheless, the evident consumer satisfaction coupled with a good safety record suggest that TENS does have a part in early labour, when labour is expected to be short, or as a complement to conventional analgesia.

Massage

Massage techniques are used by about 20% of women in labour.[1] Massage to the lower back may provide relief from backache and massage of the neck and shoulders may help to ease muscle tension which develops as a result of contraction pain. Abdominal massage using gentle outward strokes of the abdomen is also employed by some women. Many antenatal classes teach massage techniques to the partners and some midwives are qualified to give and teach massage techniques.

Mechanism of action

Massage is thought to work in several ways. It has an effect similar to that of TENS in blocking the transmission of pain impulses. It helps to relax taut muscles and probably has a psychological component too, reducing stress and anxiety and so reducing the associated muscle tension. Much of its effect comes from the soothing and comforting nature of repetition and from distraction.

Efficacy

In the survey by the National Birthday Trust[17] 90% of women who used massage said it was either good or very good. Pain may or may not be reduced but massage is often found to be very soothing and relaxing. A study on the efficacy of back massage during labour was carried out in an osteopathic Obstetric and Gynaecology Unit in Michigan, USA in 1981.[22] Five hundred mothers in labour received either osteopathic lumbar massage specifically designed for back pain in labour or massage of less appropriate areas of the back, this latter group being the controls. Eighty one per cent of women in the study group obtained relief and women in the control group received 30% more pethidine.

Acupuncture

Acupuncture is an ancient form of Chinese medicine, first mentioned in the literature in 581 BC and still widely practised in China today. The traditional teaching of acupuncture is based on the belief that life energy (chi) flows from organ to organ in the body through a network of invisible

42

flow lines or meridians (*ching-lo*). Meridians connect all tissues or organs of the body, regulate normal functions and reflect all pathological conditions. A block in a meridian is said to cause specific symptoms of illness and by inserting needles into specific acupuncture points on the skin, of which there are approximately 350, the flow of energy is restored and healing can occur.

The use of acupuncture to provide analgesia for surgery was introduced in China relatively recently, in 1958[23] and in some centres 10–30% of operations,[23-27] including elective caesarean section,[27,28] are performed using this technique. Although acupuncture in obstetrics is still practised in China, its use has declined recently with the increasing use of Western medical methods. A range of ailments during pregnancy, such as nausea, hyperemesis, backache and constipation, are treated with acupuncture.[29] A technique is described in which moxibustion is used to apply heat to an acupuncture point on the foot to convert a breech presentation to cephalic.[30] Acupuncture has mainly been used for caesarean section although it is also used with the aim of inducing labour[31-34] and augmenting, and promoting regular, uterine contractions. It has been used for pain relief in labour only over the past 20 years and mainly in the Western world. The reasons for this are unclear, but it is probably because the Chinese culture views childbirth as a physiological process which does not require analgesia. Alternatively, Chinese practitioners may feel it is ineffective for labour pain or that it is impractical to use needles in labour.

Although needles are frequently inserted to a depth of 2·5–3 cm, placement is remarkably painless. Each needle is manipulated until *teh-chi* is obtained, a feeling of warmth, numbness, distension and heaviness at the site, usually extending distally; the operator feels tightness around the needle. The traditional method is then to leave the needles undisturbed for 10–30 minutes at a time. Over the past 25 years however, newer techniques have been employed and today needles are manipulated either manually by rotating between finger and thumb and rocking to-and-fro or, more commonly, electrically, by connecting them to a low voltage electrical source and providing stimulation at a frequency of around 2–3 Hz or more (low- or high-frequency electroacupuncture). Electrical stimulation of the needles was introduced solely to replace the manual burden on the acupuncturist. In either case, sufficient stimulation must be applied to induce local reflex muscular contraction. Both manual and electrical stimulation have been employed during labour. Analgesia usually develops 10–30 minutes after the start of acupuncture.[23,24,35]

Several acupuncture points have been used to provide pain relief in labour with little uniformity. The hands, lower legs, lower abdomen, sacrum, feet and ear auricle have all been used during the first stage of labour, corresponding to those points used to treat pain of dysmenorrhoea and for caesarean section, and the upper inner thigh and perineum for the second stage.[31,35-38] As well as the traditional sites on the ancient acupuncture charts new points are constantly being used and acupuncturists may vary the points for different people.

Mechanisms of action

Despite the meridian theory having been taught for many thousands of years it has many sceptics, and even Chinese doctors accept there may be other explanations for the effects.[28] Early investigations suggested that the acupuncture point was a discrete electrical entity with electrical conductance greater than that of surrounding skin.[39-41] The success of dummy points, however, casts doubt on this (see below), and in 1972 Wall stated "there is not one scrap of anatomical or physiological evidence for the existence of such a system".[42]

Studies in the West have confirmed that acupuncture raises the pain threshold.[43,44] The mechanism remains uncertain but both the neural and hormonal systems have been suggested as likely mediators. The delay observed before the onset of analgesia and the persistent effect seen after the cessation of acupuncture[45] along with the observation that cerebrospinal fluid transferred from rabbits receiving acupuncture produced analgesia in recipient rabbits[46] all support the release of a humoral factor. One favoured mediator is β-endorphin, probably released into the cerebrospinal fluid as part of a neurohumoral mechanism. Low frequency electroacupuncture raises β-endorphin levels in the cerebrospinal fluid of patients with chronic pain[47] and naloxone reverses the analgesia of both low frequency electroacupuncture and manual acupuncture, in animals[48] and in humans experiencing pain.[49] Analgesia produced by high frequency electroacupuncture is not reversed by naloxone at normal doses and both serotonin[48,50] and met-enkephalin[51] have been proposed as mediators. Serotonin-containing pathways project from the medulla to the spinal cord and are activated by stimuli from the periaqueductal grey matter. These pathways synapse in the dorsal horns on enkephalin-containing interneurones which in turn inhibit spinal neurones mediating pain sensations.[52] A reduction in serotonin in the brain reduces the analgesic effect of high frequency but not low frequency electroacupuncture in mice.[48] Cheng and Pomeranz[48] suggested that acupuncture analgesia could be mediated by at least two pain-relieving mechanisms, one being the endorphin system which is reversed by naloxone and the other being a non-endorphin system probably involving serotonin and met-enkephalin. Acupuncture may stimulate β-endorphin-containing neurones of the periaqueductal grey matter and so stimulate endogenous pain control pathways in a manner similar to transcutaneous electrical nerve stimulation.

Neural and hormonal mechanisms probably interact. Neural conduction is obviously necessary on the afferent side since some effects of acupuncture are blocked by prior infiltration of local anaesthetic around the acupuncture point[28,53] or when the nerve is blocked proximally.[54]

A psychological component may also play a part in the success of acupuncture. Whilst it is known to raise the threshold to pain as well as to produce an area of specific analgesia, pain relief is rarely complete and the degree of hypoalgesia depends on the patient's pain threshold and psychological preparation as well as pharmacological premedication.[24]

Efficacy

Acupuncture for surgery in China is said to be successful in up to 99% of cases.[24,27,28] However, this is after careful patient selection requiring enthusiasm and acceptance of the technique, and anyone who appears tense or frightened of acupuncture receives conventional anaesthesia.[27,28] Furthermore, acupuncture for surgery is usually supplemented with opioids, local anaesthetics and sedatives.[24,26–28] In addition, the stoicism of the Chinese, indoctrination in political matters and a cultural background in which acceptance of the technique is high,[27,28] suggest a psychological element may play a part in the success of acupuncture. It is doubtful that these factors alone are adequate explanation for the success of acupuncture anaesthesia in China, but without them, results would be expected to be less satisfactory.

It is generally accepted that the greatest success with acupuncture lies in the treatment of chronic conditions such as back pain, arthritis, migraine and asthma.[24] Although the use of acupuncture in the Western world is growing slowly in these areas, many doctors, including Chinese physicians, are divided in their views on its efficacy.[24] There have been no double blind placebo-controlled, randomised clinical trials, the gold standard in determining the effects of a treatment on health. Placebo acupuncture may be achieved with needles inserted into acupuncture sites and not stimulated or placed in inappropriate sites. However, many acupuncturists believe needles inserted in non-indicated points may also confer some benefit, lending support to the argument that the meridian system does not exist. Randomisation is possible, however, but this has not been done. The difficulties encountered in designing suitable trials may account for the conflicting results obtained. All the trials examining the efficacy of acupuncture use small numbers, from which it is difficult to draw conclusions and, in addition, the skill of the acupuncturist must have some effect in determining the success rate.

A few uncontrolled or poorly controlled trials of acupuncture during labour and delivery have been reported in Western medical journals.[35–37,55,56] Overall, they do not demonstrate a significant reduction in pain scores or in the need for conventional methods of analgesia. Wallis et al[36] planned a two-part study to investigate the safety and efficacy of manual and electrical acupuncture performed by a professor from the Chinese College of Acupuncture in Hong Kong. The first part was an open study in volunteer parturients, whilst the second part was to be a controlled study of treatment and dummy-treatment groups. This part was abandoned because in the first part neither manual nor electroacupuncture provided adequate analgesia in 90% of women and 76% resorted to other forms of analgesia, though all were motivated volunteers. Yet despite these fairly negative results, one third of the women said they would have acupuncture again.

Abouleish and Depp[35] examined electroacupuncture in 12 women during childbirth. Although more than half the women obtained an average of 66% analgesia, one-third found the pain unaltered and additional analgesia was required by all but one woman. The authors concluded that analgesia was inconsistent, unpredictable and incomplete, but despite this, maternal satisfaction was high and 9 out of the 12 women said they would use it again because they remained alert, no drugs were involved and there were no side effects. One woman withdrew because she did not like the vibration of the needles and two said they would not use it again because they obtained no analgesia.

Manual acupuncture has also been used in obstetric patients with similarly disappointing and unpredictable results. In a series of 10 women analgesia was described as adequate in 10%, partial in 30% and absent in 60%.[55] In a further uncontrolled observational study, 63% of women had "adequate" analgesia whilst 37% obtained no pain relief at all.[37]

What is clear is that the effect of acupuncture on pain in labour is hugely variable. For many women there is no effect at all, whilst for others analgesia is rarely complete. However, women receiving acupuncture claim to feel calmer and more in control of their labour.[56] This and the lack of side effects may go some way to explaining why, despite the poor analgesia obtained by many women, maternal satisfaction remains fairly high.[37,56] The relative failure of acupuncture to relieve the pain of labour may even be because the wrong acupuncture points are used or because inappropriate parameters for electrical stimulation are employed. Whatever the reason, acupuncture is infrequently used in current obstetric practices in the UK.

Contraindications

Contraindications relate only to the use of electroacupuncture. It cannot be used in the bath and it interferes with electronic monitoring of the fetal heart and of the mother.

Disadvantages

There are apparently no adverse effects for the mother.[35-37] Preparation is time-consuming, with at least 2-3 sessions required before labour while the acupuncturist also needs to be present for much of labour. The sessions are expensive, often £15-£30 per preparatory session and more for the longer initial consultation plus the fee for attending labour. There is little or no pain associated with the procedure, although a few women dislike the vibrations associated with electroacupuncture.[35] The wires and equipment required for electroacupuncture limit movement and needles may become dislodged.

Effects on labour and the baby

In the absence of randomised controlled trials it is impossible to say whether acupuncture affects progress of labour or neonatal well-being, though no obvious adverse effects are reported.[35,36]

Water baths

Although bathing in warm water during labour dates back many centuries, it is only during the past 15 years that there has been renewed interest in the use of water as a therapeutic agent for labour and delivery. Most interest has centred around submerging in a bath, although water may also provide some relief as a hot shower, dabbed on the skin as a cool pad, or a hot pack such as a hot water bottle in the small of the back for backache. Promotion in the English language literature in the early 1980s and an account of an underwater delivery in the UK in a national women's magazine in 1987 precipitated a surge of interest in the water bath for labour and delivery, from both mothers and midwives. So much so, that in 1992 the House of Commons Health Committee's report on maternal services recommended that all hospitals should provide women with the option of a birthing pool wherever possible.[57] All this despite very little evidence regarding the efficacy and safety of this option for either labour or delivery.

A purpose-built water bath for use during labour needs to be large enough for the mother to change position easily and deep enough for her to submerge; dimensions commonly approximate 7 feet by 4 feet wide and up to 3 feet deep. Often made from reinforced fibreglass and insulated with foam, the bath should also be non-slip. Easy access is required from at least three sides. A form of temperature control must be incorporated into the design. Some baths have a thermostatically controlled heating system; others use a thermometer and the addition or removal of hot and cold water or a thermostatically controlled water pump. Rapid filling is needed and, more importantly, rapid emptying in case of an emergency such as cord compression. Some designs incorporate a whirlpool although concern has been expressed regarding the cleaning of these jacuzzi-style baths.[58] A cleaning protocol should be employed after each use. Simpler pools are portable and can be filled and emptied through a hose pipe.

Many people use the hot tub for its analgesic, relaxant, and soothing effects. One of the main benefits of labouring in water appears to be the feeling of buoyancy from the support given by the water. This also makes the mother more mobile and better able to change position. Women using the warm tub in labour often do so early in labour and then leave it when additional analgesia is required. Self-administered nitrous oxide is the only pharmacological analgesia that should be used in the pool; systemic opioids must be avoided because of the potential risks associated with their sedative effect.

Mechanism of action

The mechanism by which pain relief is obtained from water may be similar to that of transcutaneous electrical nerve stimulation (TENS). Sensations of warmth and pressure from the water all over the body may inhibit transmission of pain. The pleasurable sensations from warm water may also enhance the secretion of endorphins. The feel and warmth of the water is very calming and soothing to many mothers and encourages relaxation both physically and mentally, so reducing pain and helping the mother to cope with the pain. Odent[59] claimed that these effects may also reduce the secretion of endogenous catecholamines and so accelerate labour, though he reported no data.

Efficacy

There have been many anecdotal reports in support of warm water for pain relief in labour[58-62] but little well-conducted research to evaluate its true efficacy. Controlled studies provide conflicting results. Four non-randomised cohort studies have been published.[63-66] Lenstrup et al[64] demonstrated a reduction in pain score in women immersed in water. However, mean pain scores were higher before immersion than in a control group, similar 30 minutes after entering the bath and then increased similarly in both groups thereafter. Waldenström and Nilsson,[65] Burns and Greenish[63] and Busine and Guérin[66] demonstrated a reduction in the use of pharmacological analgesia. However, randomised controlled trials of labour in water have been completed by Bastide (as reported by McCandlish and Renfrew)[67] and Cammu et al,[68] and neither suggest any reduction in pain score or in use of alternative analgesia. Cammu et al found that the mean length of stay in the bath was less than one hour and the main reason for leaving it was intensified labour pain. Two large prospective randomised controlled trials are in progress to assess the efficacy of warm water more fully.[67]

In addition to pain relief, other benefits have been claimed for warm water in labour: faster cervical dilatation and shorter labour, avoidance of medical intervention, physical and mental relaxation and a better emotional experience.[58-60,62-64] The prospective randomised controlled trials by Cammu et al[68] and Bastide[67] examined these claims. Although Cammu et al found a trend towards faster cervical dilatation in the bathing group there was no difference between the two groups in labour duration. Bastide[67] found that mean duration of labour was actually longer in the bathing group than in controls. There were no differences demonstrated in operative delivery rate, perineal trauma, blood loss, neonatal condition or postpartum pyrexia.

Whatever benefits warm water may or may not have on pain or on labour progress, it elicits favourable responses from many mothers, whose satisfaction is high.[63,64,66,68] Many report that warm water has a "soothing" effect on pain and relaxes the body, particularly between contractions, and a high proportion say they will use the bath again in a future labour. Once again it is apparent that analgesic effectiveness is not a prerequisite for maternal satisfaction, which is prominent for many alternative therapies.

Contraindications

Continuous fetal heart monitoring presents a problem. Most women using the bath in labour have intermittent fetal monitoring using the Pinnard stethoscope or by hand-held Doppler but neither of these provides a printed record. Epidural analgesia is contraindicated if the mother wishes to submerge in water, although once the epidural is in place and working she rarely wishes to continue using the bath. Neither TENS nor electroacupuncture can be used in the water bath.

Use of the water bath should be restricted to uncomplicated pregnancies. Cephalo-pelvic disproportion, diabetes, cardiac disease, placenta praevia and sedative drugs are often considered to be contraindications. Pre-eclampsia is a relative contraindication. The warmth of the water may help to reduce the blood pressure in pre-eclampsia, but the effects on blood flow to the fetus are unknown. Furthermore, continuous fetal monitoring is, of course, advisable in any such condition in which the fetus is at risk.

Side effects and complications

The scarcity of formal trials means data on the benefits and risks associated with the use of water baths are lacking. Most of the potential risks associated with water baths are related to delivery under water rather than to labour in water (see below). Potential disadvantages include increased risk of infection, unrealistic or unmet expectations, restriction of choice of analgesia and restriction of mobility. The true risk of maternal infection is unknown since numbers are still small, but reports so far have been rare.[67-69] For the caregiver there is an increased risk of musculoskeletal injury[70] and blood-borne infection. Some centres now exclude women found to be HIV, hepatitis B or hepatitis C positive after mandatory screening.[71] Logistic disadvantages include unavailability of suitable pools; the mother must either obtain a pool and meet the cost of hire, or find a hospital with one.

Effects on the baby

Zimmermann et al[72] have raised concerns about the physiological changes resulting from immersion in warm water. When the water temperature is 37 °C or above there is maternal cutaneous vasodilatation and the blood is redistributed to the skin at the expense of other areas. Mean arterial blood pressure falls[73] and there is a theoretical risk of decreased placental perfusion. Furthermore, heat loss is reduced and, depending on the water temperature, heat may be transferred to the mother and fetus. The temperature of the fetus is up to 0·8 °C warmer than the mother.[74-77] Most of the heat produced by the fetus is dissipated through the placenta to the mother down the temperature gradient,[75] and a rise in maternal temperature would result in a rise in fetal temperature, which is potentially harmful,[74] through an increase in fetal basal metabolic rate and oxygen requirement, brain damage or death. Alternatively, fetal tachycardia may be misdiagnosed as fetal distress and may lead to unnecessary intervention. The optimum temperature is not known, but most sources recommend a water temperature no higher than 36–37 °C and hourly monitoring of maternal temperature.[78] Deans and Steer[78] reported five cases of fetal tachycardia which developed whist the mother laboured in a birthing pool, all of which were associated with a maternal oral temperature of between 37·5 and 38·4 °C. On leaving the pool or cooling the water all the fetal heart rates returned to normal and all the women were afebrile within 3 hours. Rosevear et al[79] reported two cases of unexpected hypoxic ischaemic encephalopathy in babies born following labour, but not delivery, in water, one of which died. They suggested that the temperature of the water *may* have been a contributing factor.

In 1983, however, Odent had suggested, without providing evidence from a randomised trial, that the fetal condition was improved by a warm bath in labour.[59] Meanwhile, others have claimed potential risks for the baby, including increased risk of infection and increased admission to the special care baby unit as well as hyperthermia.[57,65,69,70,80–82] Subsequent randomised and non-randomised controlled studies have failed to demonstrate any benefit in terms of Apgar score, neonatal stress hormones

50

or umbilical acid–base balance,[64,67,68,83] but equally, they did not detect any harmful effects. Waldenström and Nilsson,[65] in a retrospective study, reported significantly more babies with low Apgar scores born to women who had bathed than controls, but this applied only to babies born more than 24 hours after rupture of the membranes.

Water birth

Many women using the pool during labour leave it to give birth. However, delivery under water has become fashionable over the past 15 years, following numerous claims regarding benefits for both mother and baby. Underwater delivery is held to be more natural (although neither primitive humans nor primates have been known to give birth under water), and more attractive for the fetus because this is similar to the environment in the uterus. Kitzinger[58] has claimed an increase in perineal flexibility, resulting in less perineal trauma. However, Church[61] observed no difference in perineal trauma between mothers who delivered under water and those who did not, and in an unrandomised but controlled study by Burns and Greenish[63] there was a higher incidence of trauma in the bathing group.

The safety of water birth has received some bad press recently. The real risks and benefits of underwater delivery are not known, since at present the number of deliveries is too small and no large randomised controlled trials have been completed. Even with such trials, it may be difficult to pick up rare complications such as water embolus, neonatal morbidity or mortality. So far there is no evidence to suggest that water birth is either safe or unsafe. It is worrying, however, that a new practice such as water birth should be introduced without initial rigorous evaluation such as is required for the introduction of a new drug.

There have been several reports of neonatal death during uncontrolled water births.[72] In France a baby died in a home birth without an attending midwife. It was, however, held under water for nearly one hour.[84] The main risks to the baby appear to be of inhalation of water and infectious material, and of hypoxia. Kitzinger[58] claims that because of the even pressure of the water on the baby's chest the baby will not attempt to breathe under water. Odent[59] believes the baby will not breathe until triggered by contact with the air and a sudden temperature change, stating categorically "there is no risk of inhalation of water". There is little scientific evidence to support either of these claims and, moreover, both appear to overlook the baby's need for respiratory gas exchange. It is of course well recognised that babies breathe in utero, amniotic fluid passing in and out of the lungs. This process is a prerequisite for lung development. If the baby gasps under water, tap water will pass into the lungs, effectively causing fresh water drowning. Any skin flora and faecal material present

51

in the water will also be inhaled with the potential for causing infection. It is not known how long a baby can remain submerged before the oxygen supply to the brain is compromised. A popular misconception is that the baby continues to receive oxygenated blood via the umbilical cord after delivery. Pulsations felt in the cord are from the umbilical arteries and are no indication that fetal blood is being oxygenated via the placenta. After delivery the placenta usually separates, precluding oxygen exchange, so there is limited time for the baby to reach the surface and breathe. Kitzinger suggests a randomly chosen maximum of 2 minutes for submersion[58] but without any scientific evidence to support this. Approximately 4 minutes is generally allowed for a baby born in normal atmospheric conditions to take the first breath, but if a baby remains submerged and subsequently requires resuscitation, much of this leeway is lost.

Potential risks for the mother include infection, increased postpartum haemorrhage, and water embolus.[70,80] Early literature suggested that the third stage of labour should be conducted out of the water because of the risk of water embolus.[59,62] The risk of this occurrence is unknown, and many women remain in the bath for delivery of the placenta.

Summary

Although a warm bath during labour fails to provide objective pain relief for many mothers it does appear to have a soothing effect, allowing the mothers to relax, particularly between contractions. Maternal satisfaction is high and since side effects are few, it seems sensible to offer the warm tub to mothers in labour as a prelude to conventional analgesia. However, the risks of underwater delivery are undetermined and it would be prudent to exercise caution until sufficient data are available for it to be considered a safe form of birth.

Water blocks

Water blocks involve intradermal injections of approximately 0·1 ml of sterile water in four spots overlying the borders of the sacrum, usually by the attending midwife. An initial burning sensation for 20–30 seconds is all that is felt. The technique has been used in an attempt to reduce low back pain in labour[85,86] and has been particularly popular in some Scandinavian countries, but because of equivocal efficacy the technique has not become widespread.

Mechanism of action

The mechanism of action, if such there is, has been suggested to be similar to that of transcutaneous electrical nerve stimulation (see above). The local irritation caused by hypotonic sterile water injected intradermally is designed to act as a strong sensory stimulus to the surrounding skin, thought to prevent or reduce transmission of pain impulses at spinal level.

Efficacy

Some reports on the use of water blocks have demonstrated a significant reduction in labour pain,[85,86] whilst others have shown no effect.[87] Both Ader et al[85] and Trolle et al[86] compared sterile water blocks with a control group receiving a placebo intradermal injection of isotonic saline, in double blind randomised controlled studies. In both studies pain scores were reduced for up to 2 hours after the blocks in both the study and control groups, but the difference was significantly greater in the sterile water groups. However this did not result in a reduction in the need for additional analgesia. Ranta et al[87] found no reduction in pain scores following water blocks (Figure 3.3), but equally they found none following nitrous oxide or pethidine.

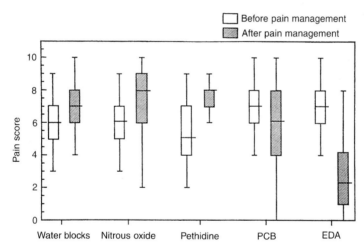

FIGURE 3.3—*Visual analogue pain scores (0–10) before and after pain management in the first stage of labour. Median values: boxes represent interquartile ranges and the whiskers, total ranges. PCB, paracervical block; EDA, epidural analgesia. (From Ranta et al[87] by permission of the author and publisher)*

Intradermal "anaesthesia"

The intracutaneous or subcutaneous infiltration with procaine hydrochloride has been tried for the relief of labour pain as far back as the

53

1920s.[88,89] Infiltration of local anaesthetic from the symphysis pubis to the anterior superior iliac spines in an arc following the lines of the inguinal ligaments, and up the midline of the abdomen was claimed to abolish abdominal pain. Infiltration over the sacrum was used to relieve back pain.

Pain relief was thought to be achieved by blocking the cutaneous branches of T10–L1 through which pain was referred to the lower abdomen and back. Pain relief was said to last approximately 3 hours, was more effective in early labour, and for abdominal rather than back pain. In observational studies both Abrams[89] and Rose[88] reported complete or very good pain relief in over 90% of women. Nevertheless this technique was never widely used and it is now purely of historical interest.

Abdominal decompression

Abdominal decompression was introduced by the South African Professor O.S. Heyns in 1955,[90] to attempt to relieve the pain of labour and to shorten its duration. He had been experimenting with suxamethonium during labour, which he noted, unexpectedly, produced rapid cervical dilatation but, not surprisingly, the respiratory impairment was a problem requiring general anaesthesia and respiratory support. Abdominal decompression was developed to mimic the beneficial effect of suxamethonium, that of relaxation of the abdominal wall musculature. The theory is that by lifting the muscles of the anterior abdominal wall off the uterus it can assume a more spherical shape, a position thought to be more conducive to efficient uterine contractions. A rigid shell or light cage covered with polythene was sealed over the lower chest, abdomen and thighs and an electrically operated suction device generated a negative pressure of 20–150 mmHg inside the shell. The suction could be controlled by the mother by occluding a hole in the connecting pipe during each contraction. Alternatively an intermittent technique of 15 seconds on, 15 seconds off was used or the suction could be maintained continuously.

Efficacy

In an uncontrolled study of 100 primiparae, Heyns reported that 91 achieved fair to complete pain relief.[90] Quinn et al[91] studied 593 women and reported excellent or good pain relief in 86%. Both Heyns[90] and Quinn et al[91] claimed a reduction in the duration of the first stage of labour. However, Heyns had no control group and Quinn selected 100 control women after delivery who had not received abdominal decompression. More recent studies[92,93] did not show it to be a successful method of pain relief, demonstrated no effect on the duration of labour and found it to be unpopular with women. In a study of 100 women Castellanos et al[93]

54

reported 53 complete failures while only 3 women obtained complete pain relief. Thirty eight women obtained some pain relief but still required additional analgesia. There is no doubt that some women have achieved considerable pain relief with abdominal decompression but it is difficult to determine how much of this was due to the decompression and how much due to a form of distraction therapy.

Heyns claimed that abdominal decompression also increased utero-placental blood flow and fetal oxygenation.[94] However, blood-gas analysis of fetal scalp capillary samples failed to support this view.[95]

Side effects and complications

The equipment is expensive and cumbersome and the electric motor used to generate the suction is noisy. The shell produces pressure on the chest, restricts limb movements, has to be removed for abdominal and vaginal examination[96] and limits fetal monitoring. Furthermore, mothers commonly lie in the supine position (Figure 3.4). Whilst decompression enjoyed a period of popularity in the 1960s, its use has virtually died out now.

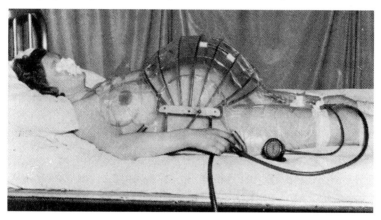

FIGURE 3.4—*Abdominal decompression apparatus. (From Scott and Loudon*[96] *by permission of the author and publisher.)*

Aromatherapy

Aromatherapy uses the essential oils of plants and flowers to alleviate certain conditions. Essential oils may be inhaled, ingested or absorbed through the skin. A few drops of oil may be placed on a pillow or handkerchief, dropped directly on to the skin or added to bath water or to creams, lotions and massage oils. A drop on a strip of absorbent card may be held by the mother or pinned to her clothing. Aromatic oils may also

55

be taken orally as diluted drops or absorbed as pessaries or suppositories.

The most common oil used in labour is lavender. It is claimed to relieve anxiety, to strengthen as well as to relax uterine contractions, to reduce pain and to have calming, sedative and relaxing properties. Clary sage is also used to speed labour by relieving stress, tension and anxiety as well as by its oestrogen-like properties. Camomile is claimed to be anti-inflammatory while jasmine and rose have antidepressant properties. Peppermint is used for nausea and vomiting.[97,98]

Putative mechanism of action   It has been suggested that the aroma of each essential oil is detected by the olfactory nerve endings in the nose acting as a trigger in a specific area of the brain to release neurochemicals with specific healing effects. For example, oils with analgesic properties may cause the release of endorphins. However, there is no scientific evidence to support or refute these claims.

Efficacy

There are no randomised controlled trials on the use of aromatherapy in childbirth and the Royal College of Obstetricians and Gynaecologists has called for a proper evaluation of the practice. In an uncontrolled study, Burns and Blamey[99] evaluated the use of ten different essential oils during labour with respect to their analgesic, anxiolytic, relaxant and antiemetic effects and their ability to stimulate uterine contractions. The women were selected as "suitable" by the midwives if they were in early or established labour, had no known allergies and wanted aromatherapy. The midwife selected the oils she/he thought most appropriate, and the method of administration. The main reason for selecting an oil was to reduce anxiety, followed by nausea, augmentation of uterine contractions and pain relief. Sixty two per cent of women described the oils as "effective" whilst 12% found them ineffective and the remainder were unsure. Only 13% required no other form of pain relief but there was a high degree of overall satisfaction on the part of the mothers and midwives.

Disadvantages

There are no reported side effects to the use of essential oils during childbirth. The main disadvantage is the cost of the oils and finding a qualified aromatherapist with an interest in childbirth.

Audioanalgesia

This rarely used technique is really one of distraction. White sound is a mixture of sounds of many frequencies, just as the colour white is a mixture of light wavelengths. It is played to the patient through earphones and is usually described as sounding similar to rushing water. The volume can be increased by the mother during contractions as the pain increases, and in between contractions soothing music may be played.

It was first used in dental practice in the 1950s and was later taken up by Burt and Korn in 1964[100] for use in obstetrics. They claimed it was useful in two-thirds of cases and that it reduced the need for pethidine. It is harmless, though it may impede communication with the mother.

Homeopathy

Homeopathy and herbalism do not strictly fall into the category of "Physical methods", but they are included here for completeness. Homeopathy has been used by the Greeks as far back as the fifth century BC. Interest was revived by a German doctor, Samuel Hahnemann, and homeopathy was introduced to England by Dr Frederick Quinn early in the nineteenth century. It works on the premise that "like cures like", homoios being the Greek word for "like with like". A disorder is treated with minute doses of a substance that in larger quantities would cause the same symptoms and signs. Substances are derived from animal, vegetable and occasionally mineral sources, and many are poisonous in large quantities.

Homeopathy is thought to act by stimulating the body's own immune system, enabling the body to heal itself. Two of the most commonly used substances for childbirth are caulophyllum and arnica. Caulophyllum is given during the later weeks of pregnancy to "tone" the uterus, and during labour to help ineffectual, exhausting uterine contractions in order to make labour easier, shorter and less painful. Arnica is claimed to reduce bruising and swelling. Several other substances are used during labour for their calming effect, to reduce pain and fatigue and to speed labour including gelsemium, kali carb, kali phos, chamomilla, bryonia, belladonna and *Bellis perennis*. Homeopathic remedies may be taken orally in tablet form, as a powder dissolved in water or as drops on the tongue.[101,102] Because homeopathy takes a holistic approach to treatment a homeopathist will customise a kit before labour, taking into account the woman's age, past medical history, temperament, food likes and dislikes and personality.

Efficacy

There is little evidence to suggest homeopathic remedies reduce pain but they may help the devotee to cope with pain, and to calm, soothe and relax her emotionally.

Herbalism

Herbalists employ the raw form of an active ingredient used by homeopathists. Each herb is believed to have its own affinity with a certain part of the body and to perform specific functions. Herbs are administered either as an infusion, in powdered form, as a capsule or as a tincture. Substances are combined so they can work together. Rosemary leaf tea is said to strengthen uterine muscles. Strawberry leaves are claimed to aid pain relief. Raspberry leaf tea, poppyhead tea and fresh coriander leaves are also associated with properties beneficial to labour[103] although no formal studies have been performed to validate these claims.

Summary

Though many non-pharmacological approaches to pain relief have been put forward, few have been widely used and fewer still subjected to randomised trials, so regrettably little rational information is available.

References

1 Steer P. The methods of pain relief used. In: Chamberlain G, Wraight A, Steer P, eds. *Pain and its relief in childbirth: the results of a national survey conducted by the National Birthday Trust.* Edinburgh: Churchill Livingstone, 1993:49–67.

2 Robson JE. Transcutaneous nerve stimulation for pain relief in labour. *Anaesthesia* 1979; **34:**357–60.

3 Stewart P. Transcutaneous nerve stimulation as a method of analgesia in labour. *Anaesthesia* 1979;**34:**361–4.

4 Shealy CN. Transcutaneous electrical stimulation for control of pain. *Clin Neurosurg* 1974;**21:**269–77.

5 Bundsen P, Peterson L-E, Selstam U. Pain relief in labor by transcutaneous electrical nerve stimulation. A prospective matched study. *Acta Obstet Gynecol Scand* 1981;**60:** 459–68.

6 Bundsen P, Ericson K, Peterson L-E, Thiringer K. Pain relief in labor by transcutaneous electrical nerve stimulation. Testing of a modified stimulation technique and evaluation of the neurological and biochemical condition of the newborn infant. *Acta Obstet Gynecol Scand* 1982;**61:**129–36.

7 Thomas IL, Tyle V, Webster J, Neilson A. An evaluation of transcutaneous electrical nerve stimulation for pain relief in labour. *Aust NZ J Obstet Gynaecol* 1988;**28:**182–9.

8 Miller Jones CMH. Transcutaneous nerve stimulation in labour. *Anaesthesia* 1980;**35:** 372–5.

9 Augustinsson L-E, Bohlin P, Bundsen P *et al.* Pain relief during delivery by transcutaneous electrical nerve stimulation. *Pain* 1977;**4:**59–65.

10 Melzack R, Schaffelberg D. Low-back pain during labor. *Am J Obstet Gynecol* 1987;**156:** 901–5.

11 Sjölund B, Terenius L, Eriksson M. Increased cerebrospinal fluid levels of endorphins after electro-acupuncture. *Acta Physiol Scand* 1977;**100:**382–4.

12 Chapman CR, Benedetti C. Analgesia following transcutaneous electrical stimulation and its partial reversal by a narcotic antagonist. *Life Sci* 1977;**21:**1645–8.

13 Sjölund BH, Eriksson MBE. The influence of naloxone on analgesia produced by peripheral conditioning stimulation. *Brain Res* 1979;**173:**295–301.

14 Harrison RF, Woods T, Shore M, Mathews G, Unwin A. Pain relief in labour using transcutaneous electrical nerve stimulation (TENS). A TENS/TENS placebo controlled study in two parity groups. *Br J Obstet Gynaecol* 1986;**93:**739–46.

15 Nesheim B-I. The use of transcutaneous nerve stimulation for pain relief during labor. *Acta Obstet Gynecol Scand* 1981;**60:**13–6.

16 Howie R. Client controlled pain relief during childbirth. *Midwives Chronicle* 1985;**98:** 294.

17 Wraight A. Coping with pain. In: Chamberlain G, Wraight A, Steer P, eds. *Pain and its relief in childbirth: the results of a national survey conducted by the National Birthday Trust.* Edinburgh: Churchill Livingstone, 1993:79–92.

18 Hughes SC, Dailey PA, Partridge C. Transcutaneous electrical nerve stimulation for labor analgesia. *Anesth Analg* 1988;**67:**S99.

19 Long DM. Fifteen years of transcutaneous electrical stimulation for pain control. *Stereotactic Funct Neurosurg* 1991;**56:**2–19.

20 Bundsen P, Ericson K. Pain relief in labor by transcutaneous electrical nerve stimulation. Safety aspects. *Acta Obstet Gynecol Scand* 1982;**61:**1–5.

21 Kubista E, Kucera H, Riss P. Die Wirkung der transkutanen nervstimulation auf den wehenschmerz. *Geburtshilfe Frauenheilkd* 1978;**38:**1079–84.

22 Bradford N, Chamberlain G. *Pain relief in childbirth.* London: Harper Collins, 1995: 192–3.

23 McIntyre JWR. Observations on the practice of anesthesia in the People's Republic of China. *Anesth Analg* 1974;**53:**107–10.

24 Wang JK. The practice of acupuncture in China. *Anesth Analg* 1974;**53:**111–12.

25 Smith AJ. Medicine in China. Best of the old and the new. *BMJ* 1974;**ii:**367–70.

26 Bonica JJ. Anesthesiology in The People's Republic of China. *Anesthesiology* 1974;**40:** 175–86.

27 Jenkins LC, Spoerel WE. Acupuncture: Canadian anesthetists report on visit to China. *Can Med Assoc J* 1974;**111:**1123–9.

28 Dimond EG. Acupuncture anesthesia. *JAMA* 1971;**218:**1558–63.

29 Yelland S. *Acupuncture in Midwifery.* Hale: Books for Midwives Press, 1996:10.

30 Cardini F, Marcolongo A. Moxibustion for correction of breech presentation: a clinical study with retrospective control. *Am J Chinese Med* 1993;**21:**133–8.

31 Tsuei JJ, Lai Y-F. Induction of labor by acupuncture and electrical stimulation. *Obstet Gynecol* 1974;**43:**337–42.

32 Kubista E, Kucera H, Müller-Tyl E. Initiating contractions of the gravid uterus through electro-acupuncture. *Am J Chinese Med* 1975;**3:**343–6.

33 Ying Y-K, Lin J-T, Robins J. Acupuncture for the induction of cervical dilatation in preparation for first-trimester abortion and its influence on HCG. *J Reprod Med* 1985; **30:**530–4.

34 Yip SK, Pang JCK, Sung ML. Induction of labor by acupuncture electro-stimulation. *Am J Chinese Med* 1976;**4:**257–65.

35 Abouleish E, Depp R. Acupuncture in obstetrics. *Anesth Analg* 1975;**54:**83–8.

36 Wallis L, Shnider SM, Palahniuk RJ, Spivey HT. An evaluation of acupuncture analgesia in obstetrics. *Anesthesiology* 1974;**41:**596–601.

37 Umeh BUO. Sacral acupuncture for pain relief in labour: initial clinical experience in Nigerian women. *Acupunct Electrother Res* 1986;**11:**147–51.

38 Yelland S. *Acupuncture in midwifery.* Hale: Books for Midwives Press, 1996:23.

39 Hyvärinen J, Karlsson M. Low-resistance skin points that may coincide with acupuncture loci. *Med Biol* 1977;**55:**88–94.

40 Reichmanis M, Marino AA, Becker RO. D.C. Skin conductance variation at acupuncture loci. *Am J Chinese Med* 1976;**4:**69–72.

41 Reichmanis M, Marino AA, Becker RO. Electrical correlates of acupuncture points. *IEEE Trans Biomed Eng* 1975;**22:**533–5.

42 Wall P. An eye on the needle. *New Scientist* 1972;**55:**129–31.

43 Andersson SA, Ericson T, Holmgren E, Lindqvist G. Electro-acupuncture. Effect on pain threshold measured with electrical stimulation of teeth. *Brain Res* 1973;**63:**393–6.

44 Chapman CR, Gehrig JD, Wilson ME. Acupuncture compared with 33 per cent nitrous oxide for dental analgesia: a sensory decision theory evaluation. *Anesthesiology* 1975;**42:** 532–7.

45 Pomeranz B, Chiu D. Naloxone blockade of acupuncture analgesia: endorphin implicated. *Life Sci* 1976;**19**:1757–62.
46 Research Group of Acupuncture Anaesthesia, Peking. The role of some neurotransmitters of brain in finger-acupuncture analgesia. *Scientia Sinica* 1974;**17**:112–30.
47 Clement-Jones V, McLoughlin L, Tomlin S, Besser GM, Rees LH, Wen HL. Increased β-endorphin but not met-enkephalin levels in human cerebrospinal fluid after acupuncture for recurrent pain. *Lancet* 1980;**ii**:946–9.
48 Cheng RSS, Pomeranz B. Electroacupuncture analgesia could be mediated by at least two pain-relieving mechanisms; endorphin and non-endorphin systems. *Life Sci* 1979; **25**:1957–62.
49 Mayer DJ, Price DD, Rafii A. Antagonism of acupuncture analgesia in man by the narcotic antagonist naloxone. *Brain Res* 1977;**121**:368–72.
50 McLennan H, Gilfillan K, Heap Y. Some pharmacological observations on the analgesia induced by acupuncture in rabbits. *Pain* 1977;**3**:229–38.
51 Clement-Jones V, McLoughlin L, Lowry PJ, Besser GM, Rees LH, Wen HL. Acupuncture in heroin addicts: changes in met-enkephalin and β-endorphin in blood and cerebrospinal fluid. *Lancet* 1979;**ii**:380–3.
52 Basbaum AI, Fields HL. Endogenous pain control mechanisms: review and hypothesis. *Ann Neurol* 1978;**4**:451–62.
53 Dundee JW, Ghaly G. Local anesthesia blocks the antiemetic action of P6 acupuncture. *Clin Pharmacol Ther* 1991;**50**:78–80.
54 Chiang CY, Chang CT, Chu HL, Yang LF. Peripheral afferent pathway for acupuncture analgesia. *Scientia Sinica* 1973;**16**:210–17.
55 Palahniuk RJ, Shnider SM, Wu SW. Acupuncture analgesia in obstetrics. *ASA Scientific Abstracts*, 1973:49–50.
56 Skelton IF, Flowerdew MW. Acupuncture and labour – a summary of results. *Midwives Chronicle* 1988;**101**:134–7.
57 House of Commons. *HC. Maternity services. Second report*. London: HMSO, 1992.
58 Kitzinger S. Sheila Kitzinger's letter from England. *Birth* 1991;**18**:170–1.
59 Odent M. Birth under water. *Lancet* 1983;**ii**:1476–7.
60 Attwood G, Lewis R. Pool rules. *Nursing Times* 1994;**90**:72–3.
61 Church LK. Water birth: one birthing center's observations. *J Nurse Midwifery* 1989;**34**: 165–70.
62 Milner I. Water baths for pain relief in labour. *Nursing Times* 1988;**84**:38–40.
63 Burns E, Greenish K. Pooling information. *Nursing Times* 1993;**89**:47–9.
64 Lenstrup C, Schantz A, Berget A, Feder E, Rosenø H, Hertel J. Warm tub bath during delivery. *Acta Obstet Gynecol Scand* 1987;**66**:709–12.
65 Waldenström U, Nilsson C-A. Warm tub bath after spontaneous rupture of membranes. *Birth* 1992;**19**:57–63.
66 Busine A, Guérin B. Le bain de dilatation: résultats obstétricaux et répercussions sur le vécu de la naissance. *Rev Méd Brux* 1987;**8**:391-7.
67 McCandlish R, Renfrew M. Immersion in water during labor and birth: the need for evaluation. *Birth* 1993;**20**:79–85.
68 Cammu H, Clasen K, Van Wettere L, Derde M-P. "To bathe or not to bathe" during the first stage of labor. *Acta Obstet Gynecol Scand* 1994;**73**:468–72.
69 George RH. Bacteria in birthing tubs [Letter]. *Nursing Times* 1990;**86**:14.
70 Alderdice F, Renfrew MJ, Marchant S *et al.* Labour and birth in water in England and Wales. *BMJ* 1995;**310**:837.
71 Ridgway GL, Tedder RS. Birthing pools and infection control [Letter]. *Lancet* 1996; **347**:1051-2.
72 Zimmermann R, Huch A, Huch R. Water birth – is it safe? *J Perinatal Med* 1993;**21**: 5–11.
73 Weston CFM, O'Hare JP, Evans JM, Corrall RJM. Haemodynamic changes in man during immersion in water at different temperatures. *Clin Sci* 1987;**73**:613–16.
74 Macaulay JH, Randall NR, Bond K, Steer PJ. Continuous monitoring of fetal temperature by noninvasive probe and its relationship to maternal temperature, fetal heart rate, and cord arterial oxygen and pH. *Obstet Gynecol* 1992;**79**:469–74.

60

75 Power GG. Biology of temperature: the mammalian fetus. *J Dev Physiol* 1989;**12:** 295–304.

76 Wood C, Beard RW. Temperature of the human foetus. *J Obstet Gynaecol Br Commonwlth* 1963;**71:**768–9.

77 Zilianti M, Cabello F, Chacón NR, Rincón CS, Salazar JR. Fetal scalp temperature during labor and its relation to acid–base balance and condition of the newborn. *Obstet Gynecol* 1983;**61:**474–9.

78 Deans AC, Steer PJ. Labour and birth in water. Temperature of pool is important [Letter]. *BMJ* 1995;**311:**390–1.

79 Rosevear SK, Fox R, Marlow N, Stirrat GM. Birthing pools and the fetus [Letter]. *Lancet* 1993;**342:**1048–9.

80 Alderdice F, Renfrew MJ, Garcia J, McCandlish R. Labour and birth in water [Letter]. *Lancet* 1993;**342:**1563.

81 Loomes SA, Finch RG. Breeding ground for bacteria [Letter]. *Nursing Times* 1990;**86:** 14–5.

82 Hawkins S. Water vs conventional births: infection rates compared. *Nursing Times* 1995; **91:**38–40.

83 Gradert Y, Hertel J, Lenstrup C, Bach FW, Christensen NJ, Rosenø H. Warm tub bath during labor. Effects on plasma catecholamine and β-endorphin-like immunoreactivity concentrations in the infants at birth. *Acta Obstet Gynecol Scand* 1987;**66:**681–3.

84 Warren S, Ballantyne A. Fears over water births as baby Noah dies. *The Sunday Times*. London, 30.09.90.

85 Ader L, Hansson B, Wallin G. Parturition pain treated by intracutaneous injections of sterile water. *Pain* 1990;**41:**133–8.

86 Trolle B, Møller M, Kronborg H, Thomsen S. The effect of sterile water blocks on low back labor pain. *Am J Obstet Gynecol* 1991;**164:**1277–81.

87 Ranta P, Jouppila P, Spalding M, Kangas-Saarela T, Hollmén A, Jouppila R. Parturients' assessment of water blocks, pethidine, nitrous oxide, paracervical and epidural blocks in labour. *Int J Obstet Anesth* 1994;**3:**193–8.

88 Rose D. Local anaesthesia in first and second stage labor. *N Engl J Med* 1929;**201:** 117–25.

89 Abrams AA. Obliteration of pain at the site of reference by intradermal infiltration anesthesia in first-stage labor. *N Engl J Med* 1950;**243:**636–40.

90 Heyns OS. Abdominal decompression in the first stage of labour. *J Obstet Gynaecol Br Emp* 1959;**66:**220–8.

91 Quinn LJ, Dorr P, Bruyere R. Experiences with abdominal decompression during labour. *J Obstet Gynaecol Br Commonwlth* 1964;**71:**934–9.

92 Shulman H, Birnbaum SJ. Evaluation of abdominal decompression during the first stage of labor. *Am J Obstet Gynecol* 1966;**95:**421–5.

93 Castellanos R, Agüero O, de Soto E. Abdominal decompression. A method of obstetric analgesia. *Am J Obstet Gynecol* 1968;**100:**924–5.

94 Heyns OS. *Abdominal Decompression*. Johannesburg: Witwatersrand University Press, 1963:65–87.

95 Newman JW, Wood EC. Abdominal decompression and foetal blood gases. *BMJ* 1967; **iii:**368–9.

96 Scott DB, Loudon JDO. A method of abdominal decompression in labour. *Lancet* 1960; **i:**1181–3.

97 Bradford N, Chamberlain G. *Pain relief in childbirth*. London: Harper Collins, 1995: 144–53.

98 *Guidelines for midwives at the John Radcliffe Maternity Unit on the use of aromatherapy for mothers on delivery suite*. 1994.

99 Burns E, Blamey C. Using aromatherapy in childbirth. *Nursing Times* 1994;**90:**54–60.

100 Burt RK, Korn GW. Audioanalgesia in obstetrics. *Am J Obstet Gynecol* 1964;**88:**361–6.

101 Bradford N, Chamberlain G. *Pain relief in childbirth*. London: Harper Collins, 1995: 160–169.

102 *Homeopathic medicine*. Boots Company PLC, Nottingham, England.

103 Tiran MD. Complementary medicine and midwifery. *Midwives Chronicle Nursing Notes* 1988:139–42.

Part Two
Systemic analgesia

4: Inhalational analgesia

Introduction

Several inhalational agents, both gaseous and volatile, have been used successfully for pain relief in labour. The earliest to be used were ether, chloroform[1] and cyclopropane,[2] followed by trichloroethylene[3-5] and methoxyflurane.[3,4,6] Enflurane,[7] isoflurane[8] and desflurane[9] are more recent additions, but only nitrous oxide[6] is currently in widespread use.

Subanaesthetic concentrations of many inhalational agents can in theory provide analgesia during labour while preserving maternal participation and without risking loss of consciousness, regurgitation or aspiration of stomach contents. In fact the competence of the upper oesophageal sphincter is well maintained under light inhalational anaesthesia, although lost under mild sedation with barbiturate or benzodiazepine.[10] All inhalational agents readily cross the placenta and the concentration in fetal blood soon approaches that of the mother. However, since these agents are excreted almost entirely through the lungs they are readily excreted from the newborn rather than relying on metabolism in an immature liver.

The periodic nature of uterine contractions lends itself to the intermittent administration of inhalational agents. During the first 30 seconds, a contraction is felt by the mother as a tightening, followed by pain. During this initial period the mother inhales the agent in order to reach analgesic concentration before pain is felt. The efficacy of inhalational analgesia depends not only on the analgesic strength of the agent but on how quickly it reaches analgesic concentration after the start of inspiration. The ideal agent for use should therefore have a low solubility in blood and rapid onset of action, with rapid equilibration between inspired and brain concentrations. A rapid offset with complete elimination between contractions would ensure cumulation did not occur. No agent fulfils these criteria completely but nitrous oxide is the best match in current use.

Ether

Ether was the first inhalational analgesic agent used for pain relief in childbirth. James Young Simpson, the professor of midwifery in Edinburgh, first documented its use in obstetrics on 19 January 1847 when it was given to a mother to deliver a dead fetus vaginally following obstructed labour. Subsequently in the USA Nathan Colley Keep described its use for normal labour and delivery when it was given on a handkerchief to Fanny Longfellow on 7 April 1847. Simpson continued to use ether during that year but found that it had several undesirable side effects. It was a potent emetic with an unpleasant pungent odour, it was irritant and explosive. Simpson's search for a newer, better agent led him to chloroform.

Chloroform

David Waldie, a Liverpool chemist, recommended chloroform to James Young Simpson who subsequently administered it to a labouring woman on 8 November 1847. It had several advantages over ether. It had a pleasant odour, was non-irritant, more potent and faster acting and its use rapidly superseded that of ether. Simpson administered it by dropping half a teaspoonful on to a damp handkerchief rolled into the shape of a funnel and placing the open end over the woman's mouth and nose. Later the National Birthday Trust raised money for chloroform to be made up in measured doses in glass ampoules which could be emptied onto gauze placed on the patient's face.

Use of chloroform spread rapidly in the UK despite opposition to the use of pain relief in labour. There was a strong body of opinion who believed pain was a necessary and integral part of labour and to remove it meant loss of a valuable guide to the progress of labour. In addition there were worries over its safety and objections on religious grounds. The Anglican clergy condemned the technique because they believed it ran contrary to the wishes of the Creator; Genesis 3:16 states, "in sorrow thou shalt bring forth children". However chloroform received the royal seal of approval when Dr John Snow administered it from a handkerchief to Queen

Victoria for the birth of Prince Leopold, on 7 April 1853, and for the subsequent and last two of her ten children.

However, despite the initial popularity of chloroform in both general anaesthesia and midwifery, it soon became clear that the advantages offered over ether were overshadowed by its undesirable, dose-related side effects, namely arrhythmias and liver damage. Chloroform reduced the strength of uterine contractions and, like all volatile anaesthetic agents, it crossed the placenta and caused neonatal depression. When compared with the impressive safety record of ether a swing back towards the use of ether for general anaesthesia began. Its use in midwifery persisted, however, since the risk of fatal overdose was considered minimal from the lower analgesic doses given by intermittent inhalation. Yet administration was uncontrolled and analgesia frequently progressed to anaesthesia. Its use declined until the Tecota chloroform inhaler was developed to provide a measured concentration thus improving its safety. Until the mid-1950s chloroform was really the only effective pharmacological analgesic agent used in labour, although by today's standards it was not widely used. It was superseded by nitrous oxide.

Nitrous oxide

History

Nitrous oxide is the only inhalational agent in frequent use today for the relief of pain in labour. It is one of the most popular forms of pain relief, available in 99% of units in the UK and used by 60% of women in labour.[11] It was introduced into obstetric practice in 1880 by Klikovicz and has been in widespread use since the 1930s. Initially it was administered by an anaesthetist who adjusted the concentrations of nitrous oxide and air from separate sources. In 1933 Dr R J Minnitt developed a system for its premixing.[12] The Minnitt gas and air analgesia apparatus permitted for the first time the administration of an analgesic drug by unsupervised midwives. Initially a 50:50 mixture with air was used but in 1962 Cole and Nainby-Luxmoore discovered that in some cases women were breathing as little as 8% oxygen.[13] So oxygen was substituted for air and administered via the Minnitt or Lucy Baldwin apparatus. These machines were cumbersome and not readily portable but initially it was not considered possible to mix the two agents in one cylinder since oxygen is stored as a gas and nitrous oxide as a liquid. However in 1961 Tunstall demonstrated that under a pressure of 2000 p.s.i. oxygen would dissolve nitrous oxide in the gas phase producing a mixture that behaves as a single gas.[14] Since then this mixture has been marketed as Entonox by the British Oxygen Company.

67

Physical and chemical properties

Nitrous oxide is a fast acting inhalational agent. It has a low potency (MAC 105) but good analgesic properties in subanaesthetic concentrations. Its low blood/gas solubility coefficient (Table 4.1) allows rapid equilibration

TABLE 4.1—*Characteristics of inhalational agents*

	Boiling point (°C)	Blood/gas sol. coeff. at 37 °C	Biodegradation (%)	MAC (%)
Nitrous oxide	−88	0·47	0	105
Trichloroethylene	87	9·0	20–30	0·17
Methoxyflurane	105	13·0	50–70	0·16
Enflurane	56	1·9	2·4	1·68
Isoflurane	49	1·4	<0·2	1·15
Desflurane	23	0·42	<0·1	6·0

sol. coeff., solubility coefficient.

of arterial concentration with the inspired concentration of nitrous oxide. Rapid elimination of nitrous oxide from the lungs between contractions means that, unlike methoxyflurane and trichloroethylene, it accumulates little in fetal and maternal tissues.

At temperatures above −8 °C Entonox is a gas. Below this temperature the two gases tend to separate into layers,[15,16] with gaseous oxygen on the top and the liquid nitrous oxide falling to the bottom. If the cylinder is upright the gas given off from the top consists mainly of oxygen with a low concentration of nitrous oxide. It then becomes increasingly hypoxic towards the bottom. In 1970 Cole *et al*[17] made several recommendations on the handling and storage of premixed cylinders to avoid such an occurrence. The 2000 litre cylinder, mounted on a trolley for hospital use, and the 5000 litre cylinder for connection to a hospital pipeline installation should be stored horizontally for 24 hours before use, at a temperature between 10 °C and 45 °C. During delivery to the point of use they should not be exposed to freezing temperatures for more than 10 minutes. The 500 litre cylinder for domestic use should be stored at a temperature greater than 10 °C for two hours before use, or may be warmed in a bath at body temperature for five minutes. The cylinder should be inverted gently three times before use to ensure adequate mixing. Keeping the cylinder horizontal reduces the degree of separation and therefore the risk of delivering an oxygen-deficient or nitrous oxide-deficient mixture.

Methods of administration

Entonox is self-administered from a pressurised cylinder via a reducing valve and a demand valve assembly, through a face mask or mouth piece (Figures 4.1, 4.2). Parturients are taught to start inhaling when they first

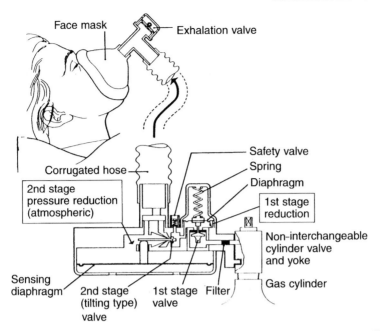

FIGURE 4.1—*Pressure reducing valve in the Entonox apparatus. (From Doughty*[18] *by permission of the author and publisher)*

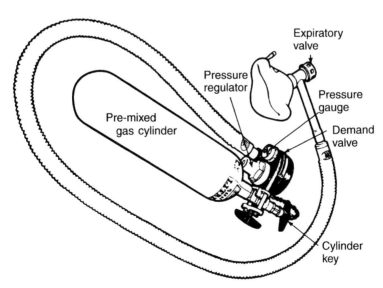

FIGURE 4.2—*The Entonox apparatus. (From Plantevin*[19] *by permission of the author and publisher)*

69

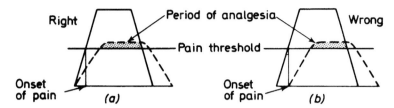

FIGURE 4.3—*The analgesic effect of 50:50 nitrous oxide and oxygen. (a) Inhalation started with onset of contraction. (b) Inhalation started with onset of pain. Nitrous oxide concentration in blood ------; uterine contraction ———. (From Plantevin[19] by permission of the author and publisher)*

feel the contraction rather than waiting until the contraction becomes painful, and to stop once the peak has passed. However, it takes 15–20 seconds to reach an effective arterial concentration of nitrous oxide, and approximately 45–60 seconds to maximum analgesic effect.[20] This is often longer than the painless period of the contraction (up to 30 seconds), so peak nitrous oxide concentration occurs after the time of maximal pain is reached[21] (Figure 4.3). Near complete elimination occurs between contractions so timing is crucial for effective pain relief. Effective use of Entonox during the second stage of labour is even more difficult. The woman should take two or three deep inhalations with the onset of the contraction followed by pushing. When the head is crowning, rapid shallow breaths of Entonox may be taken.

Faulty equipment may allow dilution of the gas through a leak in the tubing or valve or an ill-fitting face mask, and inadequate pain relief can result. A sticking valve may produce resistance to expiration, and dirty equipment may lead to infection.

Efficacy

The use of 50% nitrous oxide in oxygen is based on early trials[22-24] that examined different concentrations of nitrous oxide and found 50% to be the best compromise between analgesia, which increases at higher concentrations, and conscious level, which decreases. Using continuous inhalation of nitrous oxide, Jones et al[25] found that the optimum balance of analgesia against level of consciousness was achieved when a concentration of 41·2% was administered, and he calculated that to achieve this concentration using intermittent inhalation 74% nitrous oxide would need to be inspired.[6] McAneny and Doughty[22] studied concentrations of 50–80% nitrous oxide in oxygen by intermittent inhalation. Seventy per cent provided more effective analgesia than either 50% or 60% and at concentrations above 70% more women lost consciousness. Trials organised by the Medical Research Council[23] published in 1970 compared nitrous

TABLE 4.2—*Analgesia obtained by women using Entonox*

	Complete (%)	Satisfactory or considerable (%)	Slight (%)	None (%)
Rosen et al[4]	11	61	25	3
Holdcroft and Morgan[26]	4	46	18	30
Cole et al[23]		75% Complete or good		25% Fair or poor

oxide 50%, 60% and 70% with oxygen. Whilst similar pain relief was achieved a small but significant number of women breathing 70% became unconscious or difficult to manage (2·9% compared with 0·4% breathing Entonox). An even earlier study showed that when 85% nitrous oxide was breathed with oxygen, almost half of the women became partially anaesthetised and difficult to control.[24] In view of these findings and the fact that some women tend to inhale nitrous oxide continuously if unsupervised, the committee of the Medical Research Council concluded that a 50:50 mixture of nitrous oxide and oxygen generally provided adequate pain relief for normal delivery and could be used safely by unsupervised midwives.

Trials and surveys examining the analgesic efficacy of Entonox give mixed results.[4,26,27] It rarely relieves all the pain and has little effect on severe labour pain. Its analgesic effects have ranged between "complete" and "no analgesia" (Table 4.2). In an early trial by Rosen et al,[4] 72% of women reported complete or considerable pain relief. However, Holdcroft and Morgan[26] reported satisfactory analgesia in only 46% of women, 30% received no pain relief and only 4% found analgesia complete. Early trials by Cole et al,[23] which were supported by the Medical Research Council, found similarly disappointing results, with 25% of women claiming inadequate analgesia with 50% nitrous oxide. However, surveys show that it is generally better than pethidine and TENS.[26,28,29] In the National Birthday Trust survey,[28] 43% of women using Entonox identified it as helpful in the relief of pain compared with 28% using pethidine and 22% using TENS, while 13% of women rated Entonox as unhelpful compared with 14% pethidine and 20% TENS. Similarly, Harrison et al[29] demonstrated success with Entonox as a primary method of pain relief in 95% of women, compared with 20% for pethidine and TENS. Satisfactory pain relief with Entonox is unrelated to parity.[26] It is often used in combination with other forms of pain relief, such as pethidine and non-pharmacological methods. However, Holdcroft and Morgan[26] showed that analgesia was not improved when pethidine was administered with nitrous oxide.

A more recent randomised, double-blind, cross-over, placebo-controlled trial by Carstoniu et al[30] compared Entonox with compressed air. Pain scores rated over five contractions were nearly identical and independent of whether the woman was breathing Entonox or compressed air (Figure

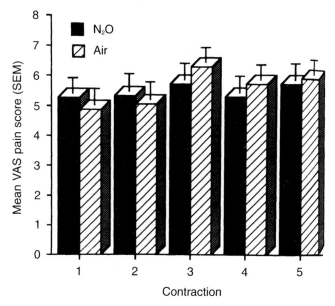

FIGURE 4.4—*Effect of nitrous oxide and air on mean visual analogue scale (VAS) pain scores during five consecutive uterine contractions. There was no difference in the VAS whether breathing nitrous oxide or air. (From Carstoniu et al[30] by permission of the author and publisher)*

4.4). The methodology of the study was superior to that of previous studies. This result is rather disappointing in view of the fact that nitrous oxide appears to be the second best analgesic for labour and yielded favourable comments in the National Birthday Trust survey.[28]

Although pain relief from Entonox depends largely on reaching an effective analgesic concentration, the distraction it can provide, the sleepiness and relaxation between contractions and the need to concentrate on the breathing may also play a part. As it is self-administered, women feel they have some control over their own pain relief.

Enhancing the effect of nitrous oxide

Much of the efficacy of nitrous oxide depends on the timing of inhalation which determines the concentration of nitrous oxide in arterial blood during the contraction, so it is helpful for mothers to be taught the technique for using Entonox before the onset of labour. The duration of pain felt can be reduced if inhalation starts when the contractions are first palpable[31] rather than when they are sensed by the mother, and analgesia can be improved further if inhalation starts before the contraction begins.[20,21] The periods between contractions need to be timed by the midwife or partner and the contractions must be regular. Although these methods ensure maximum analgesic concentrations of nitrous oxide during the contraction they are not very practical and are rarely used.

To try to reduce the need for accurate timing low concentrations of nitrous oxide have been administered continuously via a nasal catheter or prongs in both volunteers[32] and parturients.[33,34] End-tidal nitrous oxide concentration is maintained between contractions so the time to reach an effective analgesic concentration is reduced. Arthurs and Rosen[33] compared analgesia during intermittent Entonox alone and supplemented by the continuous administration of 5 l/min nasal oxygen and then Entonox, each mother acting as her own control. Nasal Entonox helped to maintain mean end-tidal nitrous oxide concentrations between contractions. No mothers lost consciousness, better pain relief was achieved and 66% preferred the nasal Entonox to nasal oxygen, but at the expense of a slight increase in sedation. However, the increase in analgesic efficacy was small as there was no difference in the use of pethidine between the two groups. Furthermore, in a larger "acceptance" study[35] of more than 1000 women, pain scores, whilst showing a trend in favour of nasal Entonox, were not significantly different, probably because the study period included the whole time up until delivery rather than just a defined period in the first stage of labour.

Analgesia may be enhanced by the addition of a volatile agent.[36,37] Levack and Tunstall[36] suggested that efficacy was improved when trichloroethylene was used to supplement 50% nitrous oxide but this combination was never available for use by unsupervised midwives. Arora et al[37] showed that intermittent inhalation of isoflurane 0·25% in Entonox gave significantly better analgesia than Entonox alone in the first stage of labour. There was a high acceptance rate, maternal cooperation was maintained and 14 out of 16 mothers chose to continue its use until delivery after the study was completed. The other two did not because they found the effect "too strong". Wee et al[38] supplemented Entonox with 0.2% isoflurane for intermittent use during labour and found a high acceptance rate and significantly lower pain scores than with Entonox alone. Although drowsiness was slightly increased it was not clinically significant. No amnesia was reported.

Side effects and complications

Many mothers feel light-headed when breathing Entonox and with prolonged use some women become drowsy, confused, drunk and disorientated; 0·4% become unconscious.[23] Nausea and vomiting are relatively common.[23]

The use of Entonox may encourage mothers to hyperventilate during contractions in an attempt to improve analgesia.[39] This may lead to symptoms of hypocapnia after prolonged use, namely dizziness, tingling and tetany. Maternal alkalosis produces a left shift of the haemoglobin–oxygen dissociation curve and vasoconstriction with a reduction in uterine blood flow,[40] both of which, potentially, reduce fetal oxygenation.[41]

There has been much debate about the effect of nitrous oxide on maternal oxygenation. Episodes of hypoxaemia occur during painful labour.[42,43] Huch et al[44] outlined the mechanism whereby the pain of uterine contractions stimulates hyperventilation thus reducing P_{CO_2}. This reduces ventilatory drive and subsequent hypoventilation or apnoea between contractions may result in maternal oxygen desaturation. During pregnancy functional residual capacity is reduced and minute ventilation and oxygen consumption are increased,[45] so hypoventilation results in hypoxia and hypercarbia more readily. The increased oxygen consumption of painful labour exacerbates this further. These episodes are potentially harmful to the fetus, not only from maternal hypoxaemia but because of the reduced oxygen delivery to the fetus consequent on maternal alkalosis. It has been suggested that Entonox may exacerbate these episodes of maternal hypoxaemia,[46–48] but none of the studies can say conclusively that Entonox alone exacerbates maternal hypoxaemia over and above that seen in normal, painful labour. For example, in a study by Lin et al[46] the control group received epidural analgesia even though epidurals have been shown to reduce the incidence of hypoxaemia compared with no analgesia[43] by removing the pain and hyperventilation. In other studies co-administration of opioids may have contributed to maternal hypoxia.[47,48] In a recent double-blind, randomised, cross-over study by Carstoniu et al[30] and an earlier study by Davies et al[49] no increase in maternal hypoxaemia was found with Entonox alone. However, in a study by Wilkins et al[50] examining the effects of Entonox on oxygenation in 10 healthy volunteers, each subject inhaled sequentially Entonox followed by 50% and 79% nitrogen in oxygen, with periods of resting ventilation and hyperventilation with each gas mixture. During the periods following resting ventilation and hyperventilation the fall in S_{PO_2} was significantly greater with Entonox, suggesting there may have been altered respiratory drive or diffusion hypoxia. Be that as it may, there appears to be little detriment for either mother or baby (see below, Effects on the baby).

Nitrous oxide is the safest inhalational agent available with no toxic actions on the heart, liver or kidneys. However, nitrous oxide interferes with methionine synthase activity by inactivating its cofactor vitamin B_{12}. One of the products of this reaction is tetrahydrofolate, a co-enzyme in the

74

biosynthesis of deoxyribonucleic acid (DNA), hence the subsequent effects of vitamin B_{12} inactivation are potentially far-reaching. Prolonged use of nitrous oxide has been associated with bone marrow suppression following the demonstration of pancytopenia and megaloblastic bone marrow changes in critically ill patients.[51,52] A demyelinating condition resembling subacute combined degeneration of the cord, usually seen in patients with vitamin B_{12} deficiency, has also been observed.[53] The doses received during labour are much less and there is no evidence to suggest that parturients or neonates are at risk from these effects.

It has been postulated that babies born to mothers treated with Entonox in labour have an increased risk of developing drug addiction in later life,[54,55] and an imprinting method was suggested. However, these retrospective studies have been heavily criticised and further studies are needed to confirm or refute these claims.

Dry gases from cylinders encourage vapour loss in expiration and with prolonged use women may suffer dry mouth and dehydration, particularly if using a mouth piece. This is exacerbated by excessive hyperventilation and a low oral fluid intake. The use of a nasal catheter or prongs for the continuous administration of Entonox to mothers in labour[33] allows humidification of the inhaled gases in the nose which is not possible when a mouthpiece is used.

Entonox cylinders are heavy and need to be transported for home delivery. Portable cylinders contain 500 litres of Entonox. Mean estimates of Entonox usage range from 290 litres for multips to nearly 800 litres in primips with uncomplicated labours,[56] so two cylinders would be needed for a multiparous home delivery and three for a nullipara.

Effects on labour

There is no evidence that nitrous oxide depresses uterine activity or prolongs labour.[57]

Effects on the baby

Although the passage of nitrous oxide across the placenta is rapid, Entonox has no known clinically significant side effects for the fetus or newborn,[58,59] since excretion through the lungs is rapid. The oxygen enrichment of the inspired gas may be helpful, although probably only when there is fetal distress. In a situation requiring an increased inspired oxygen concentration administration should be continuous rather than intermittent. Even though maternal hypoxaemic episodes occur, they have rarely been shown to be harmful to the baby as indicated by Apgar scores, Neurologic and Adaptive

Capacity Score or cord blood acid–base and gas status. The National Birthday Trust survey[60] found no greater incidence of low Apgar scores in babies born after Entonox than after no analgesia.

Other gaseous agents

An ethylene and oxygen mixture was first used in 1923 to provide analgesia in labour. Cyclopropane was also introduced at around the same time and both agents were popular, particularly in the USA. At the time when nitrous oxide was being given in concentrations greater than 50% these two potent agents were effective at lower concentrations, permitting higher inhaled concentrations of oxygen, so minimising the risk of maternal and fetal hypoxia. However, the equipment was expensive, sedation was common, interfering with pushing during the second stage of labour, and loss of consciousness occurred in some women. Cyclopropane in particular caused neonatal depression. Nitrous oxide eventually superseded them.

Trichloroethylene

Synthesised in 1864, trichloroethylene (Trilene) was introduced into obstetrics in 1943 and soon became more popular than the more toxic chloroform. It had a high boiling point (see Table 4.1) and therefore low volatility, but it had a high potency to compensate and was a good analgesic at subanaesthetic concentrations. Concentrations of 0·35–0·5% that were used for labour provided similar analgesia to 50% nitrous oxide and 0·35% methoxyflurane.[4] It had a high blood-gas solubility coefficient (see Table 4.1), conferring both advantages and disadvantages. It had a delayed onset of action but the delayed elimination meant that analgesia improved with successive contractions (Figure 4.5). Similarly, the timing of inhalation to coincide with the painless onset of each contraction was less crucial than with nitrous oxide. The mother tended, however, to become progressively drowsy. Trichloroethylene was associated with a high incidence of nausea and vomiting.[3,4] A small percentage was metabolised in the liver (see Table 4.1), but unlike with the fluorinated ethers, no hepatic or renal toxicity was observed. Trichloroethylene crossed the placenta freely and caused neonatal depression if used for longer than about an hour.[62]

Trichloroethylene was administered initially from an uncompensated draw-over vaporiser, so that women occasionally received a relative overdose causing tachypnoea, respiratory depression and arrhythmias. The accurately calibrated, temperature-compensated, draw-over vaporisers, the Emotril and Tecota Mark 6 inhalers, were developed in 1949 and 1952 respectively following standards set by the Medical Research Council to ensure accurate

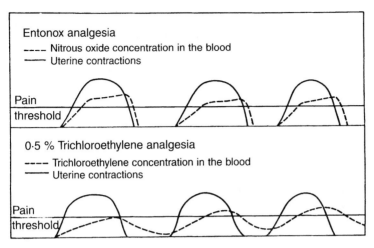

FIGURE 4.5—*A diagrammatic representation of the analgesic actions of nitrous oxide and trichloroethylene. Nitrous oxide rapidly reaches analgesic concentrations in the blood and the concentration falls rapidly between contractions. In contrast the concentration of trichloroethylene rises more slowly and does not fall to zero between contractions so trichloroethylene tends to accumulate in blood and tissues. (From Moir[61] by permission of the author and publisher)*

administration of volatile agents and to avoid potentially fatal overdose. These modified vaporisers were more accurate, ensuring concentrations of either 0·35% or 0·5% were given in air with the potential for adding oxygen to the inspired mixture. They were small, light, and readily portable. Trichloroethylene was used extensively by midwives between 1955 and 1984. Approval for its use by midwives was withdrawn by the Central Midwives Board in 1993. As a result trichloroethylene is no longer used for pain relief in labour and, indeed, has not been manufactured in the UK since 1988.

Indications and contraindications

In the days when nitrous oxide was administered in air (see above), such a reduced inspired oxygen concentration was considered to be contraindicated in cardiac or respiratory disease, which were therefore considered to be indications for the use of trichloroethylene. Hence with the advent of Entonox, the need for trichloroethylene declined.

Methoxyflurane

Methoxyflurane (Penthrane) was a halogenated ether that was introduced in 1960 in the hope that it would be superior in terms of speed of onset and elimination. This proved not to be the case. It enjoyed a brief and

77

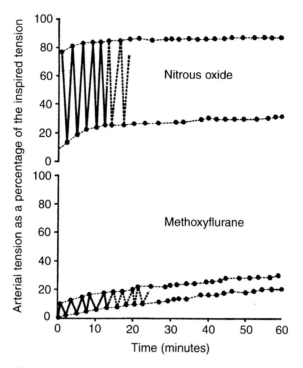

FIGURE 4.6—*Blood concentrations of nitrous oxide and methoxyflurane (provisional computed uptake) over time during intermittent inhalation. Methoxyflurane concentration increases more slowly than nitrous oxide during each contraction. It also falls more slowly, does not reach zero between contractions and so accumulation occurs over time, improving analgesia. (From Jones et al[6] by permission of the author and publisher)*

limited vogue for analgesia in labour. After extensive trials in the UK,[3,6,25] it was approved by the Central Midwives Board for self-administered analgesia during labour in 1970 (England and Wales) and 1972 (Scotland). Like trichloroethylene it had a high boiling point and low volatility (see Table 4.1), was non-explosive under the conditions used and was a potent anaesthetic (MAC 0·16) and a powerful analgesic agent. Methoxyflurane 0·35% in air was given via the Cardiff Penthrane Inhaler, a temperature-compensated, accurately calibrated draw-over vaporiser. Like trichloro-ethylene, methoxyflurane had a high blood-gas solubility coefficient (see Table 4.1) and therefore took longer than nitrous oxide to produce initial analgesia (3–4 minutes), but accumulation occurred with prolonged use and so analgesia improved over time (Figure 4.6).[6,20,21] Although it was popular in the USA, it was never as popular as trichloroethylene in the UK.

Fears over long-term renal damage eventually led to the withdrawal of methoxyflurane in 1984. High-output renal failure after prolonged methoxyflurane *anaesthesia* has been reported,[63-69] and evidence suggests this was related to the concentration of serum inorganic fluoride ions[70] released during hepatic metabolism. Intermittent inhalation of methoxyflurane in labour resulted in peak fluoride ion concentrations well below the level even for subclinical nephrotoxicity.[71] However, although the risk of clinically significant nephrotoxicity was extremely remote using methoxyflurane in labour, hepatitis was reported[72] and the availability of a safe, equally efficacious alternative in nitrous oxide eventually led to the withdrawal of methoxyflurane.

Methoxyflurane crossed the placenta and caused neonatal depression after prolonged use.[73] Although serum inorganic fluoride ion concentrations were raised in the neonate after delivery[71] the concentrations reached were well below those at which clinical nephrotoxicity would be expected.

Enflurane and isoflurane

Like methoxyflurane, enflurane and isoflurane are halogenated ethers. Both agents have been used in subanaesthetic concentrations alone or in combination with nitrous oxide for pain relief in labour. Enflurane was used for a short while during the 1980s but because of the long-term drowsiness it produced it was never very popular. Like methoxyflurane and trichloroethylene, these volatile agents are given via a draw-over vaporiser and are usually mixed with oxygen rather than air.

The main problem with the use of earlier volatile agents for pain relief in labour was their high degree of solubility in blood. Because both isoflurane and enflurane have blood-gas solubility coefficients that lie between those of nitrous oxide and both trichloroethylene and methoxyflurane (see Table 4.1), rates of uptake and elimination are faster and accumulation with intermittent inhalation is less than with methoxyflurane and trichloroethylene. Yet sufficient "carry-over" occurs from one contraction to the next so, in theory, analgesia early in the contraction should be better than with nitrous oxide. They are biodegraded less than methoxyflurane[74,75] (see Table 4.1), resulting in lower concentrations of fluoride ions,[70,76,77] particularly with isoflurane, and no evidence of organ toxicity at analgesic doses.[7,8] They can be administered in high concentrations of oxygen.

Efficacy

The use of subanaesthetic doses of enflurane and isoflurane has been examined during both the first and second stages of labour, by intermittent or continuous administration.[7,8,58,78,79] Both enflurane 1%[78] and isoflurane 0·75%[79] given by intermittent inhalation during the first stage of labour have produced better analgesia than nitrous oxide 50%, but this is at the expense of more maternal sedation. Maternal satisfaction is high; 70% of women in one study[79] said they preferred 0·75% intermittent isoflurane in oxygen whereas 25% preferred nitrous oxide. Enflurane 0·25–1·25%[7,58] and isoflurane 0·2–0·7%[8] in oxygen have been given continuously for the second stage of labour during normal vaginal delivery, but analgesia and patient satisfaction were no better than with nitrous oxide.

Ideally what is needed is a rapidly acting analgesic with rapid reversal, greater potency and efficacy than nitrous oxide and no maternal sedation. Supplementing Entonox with low concentrations of isoflurane or enflurane goes some way to providing this. The efficacy of 50% nitrous oxide is improved whilst the excessive drowsiness seen with the volatile agents alone is reduced by using lower concentrations.

Wee et al[38] and Arora et al[37] used draw-over vaporisers to supplement Entonox with isoflurane. Tunstall and Ross[80] reported, however, that isoflurane at low concentration mixed with oxygen and nitrous oxide formed a stable and constant gas mixture at cylinder pressures of 137 atmospheres and higher, and this could be self-administered through a demand valve, thus avoiding the need for a clumsy draw-over vaporiser.

Side effects and complications

Drowsiness is similar with enflurane and isoflurane and greater than with Entonox.[78,79] It is dose-related but self-limiting to a certain extent when self-administered and breathing air between the contractions.

There is the theoretical risk of renal failure from fluoride ions released during enflurane, and to a lesser extent isoflurane, metabolism. Following enflurane anaesthesia Mazze et al[76] found elevated inorganic fluoride concentrations associated with a mild reduction in urine concentrating ability, but this was after a mean enflurane exposure of 10 MAC hours. Most surgery is associated with a lower exposure, only a slight increase in serum inorganic fluoride concentration, and no renal toxicity.[81] Furthermore, no significant elevation of serum fluoride ion concentrations or impairment in renal function have been demonstrated with isoflurane or enflurane in doses used for labour analgesia.[7,8]

Occasional amnesia for the period of use has been reported[7] but use of low concentrations minimises this. Both agents have a pungent odour which may limit patient acceptance. Both are expensive and since neither shows a significant advantage over Entonox in terms of analgesia they are unlikely to be widely used on their own.

Effects on labour

Although a dose-related decrease in uterine tone has been demonstrated during anaesthesia with enflurane and isoflurane, subanaesthetic doses have not been shown to affect progress of labour or blood loss after delivery.[7,8]

Effects on the baby

Following analgesic concentrations of enflurane and isoflurane no depressant effects on the newborn have been demonstrated using Apgar scores, neurobehavioural scores and umbilical acid–base status.[7,8,58]

Desflurane

Desflurane is the newest volatile agent to be applied for analgesia in labour. Its low blood-gas partition coefficient (see Table 4.1) allows rapid onset and offset of action.

Efficacy

Desflurane in concentrations of 1–4·5% in oxygen has been compared with 30–60% nitrous oxide in oxygen during the second stage of labour.[9] Both agents were reported to be remarkably effective; more than 60% of women were reported to have little or no pain. However, there was a 23% incidence of amnesia for the delivery in the desflurane group compared with none in the nitrous oxide group. Blood loss, Apgar scores and other indices of neonatal welfare were similar.

Disadvantages

Desflurane has a low boiling point near to room temperature (see Table 4.1) and therefore requires a modified vaporiser. It is expensive and since it has not been shown to provide superior analgesia to Entonox it is unlikely to become a popular agent for labour analgesia. Furthermore, the high incidence of amnesia would be considered unacceptable by many women.

Pollution

One of the main drawbacks to the use of inhalational agents on the delivery suite is air pollution. Chronic exposure of health care workers to inhalational agents has been associated with potentially adverse effects on health.[82] Fetotoxicity and teratogenesis in rats have been claimed[83–86] and early epidemiological studies suggested an association between health problems and exposure to inhalational anaesthetics, particularly an increased incidence of spontaneous abortion in humans.[87] However, a prospective epidemiological study of 11,000 female doctors in the UK was carried out over a 10 year period (1977–87) by Spence and Knill-Jones and, though the full results were not published, it appears that no significant occupational health risk was detected.[88,89]

Despite current opinion favouring the overall safety of inhalational anaesthetic agents, in 1996 the Health and Safety Executive introduced occupational exposure standards.[90] Current standards in the UK require that ambient concentrations should not exceed 100 ppm for nitrous oxide and 50 ppm for isoflurane. However, the standard for nitrous oxide may prove difficult to meet without the use of adequate scavenging, a particular problem in the delivery suite. Although mean concentrations of nitrous oxide in theatre are generally below 400 ppm, falling to well below 100 ppm with active scavenging,[91] levels in dental surgeries of up to 6800 ppm have been detected.[92,93] In a recent study by Mills et al,[94] levels of nitrous oxide exposure in midwives frequently exceeded the new standard.

References

1 Moya F. Use of a chloroform inhaler in obstetrics. *N Y State J Med* 1961;**61**:421–9.
2 Shnider SM, Moya F, Thorndike V, Bossers A, Morishima H, James LS. Clinical and biochemical studies of cyclopropane analgesia in obstetrics. *Anesthesiology* 1963;**24**:11–17.
3 Major V, Rosen M, Mushin WW. Methoxyflurane as an obstetric analgesic: a comparison with trichloroethylene. *BMJ* 1996;**ii**:1554–61.
4 Rosen M, Mushin WW, Jones PL, Jones EV. Field trial of methoxyflurane, nitrous oxide, and trichloroethylene as obstetric analgesics. *BMJ* 1969;**iii**:263–7.
5 Gordon RA, Morton MV. Trichloroethylene in obstetrical analgesia and anaesthesia. *Anesthesiology* 1951;**12**:680–7.
6 Jones PL, Rosen M, Mushin WW, Jones EV. Methoxyflurane and nitrous oxide as obstetric analgesics. II. – A comparison by self-administered intermittent inhalation. *BMJ* 1969;**iii**:259–62.
7 Abboud TK, Shnider SM, Wright RG *et al.* Enflurane analgesia in obstetrics. *Anesth Analg* 1981;**60**:133–7.
8 Abboud TK, Gangolly J, Mosaad P, Crowell D. Isoflurane in obstetrics. *Anesth Analg* 1989;**68**:388–91.
9 Abboud TK, Swart F, Zhu J, Donovan MM, Peres Da Silva E, Yakal K. Desflurane analgesia for vaginal delivery. *Acta Anaesth Scand* 1995;**39**:259–61.
10 Vanner RG. Mechanisms of regurgitation and its prevention with cricoid pressure. *Int J Obstet Anesth* 1993;**2**:207–15.
11 Steer P. The methods of pain relief used. In: Chamberlain G, Wraight A, Steer P, eds. *Pain and its relief in childbirth: the results of a national survey conducted by the National Birthday Trust.* Edinburgh: Churchill Livingstone, 1993:49–67.
12 Minnitt RJ. Self-administered analgesia for the midwifery of general practice. *Br J Anaesth* 1934;**11**:148–52.
13 Cole PV, Nainby-Luxmoore RC. Respiratory volumes in labour. *BMJ* 1962;**i**:1118.
14 Tunstall ME. Obstetric analgesia. The use of a fixed nitrous oxide and oxygen mixture from one cylinder. *Lancet* 1961;**ii**:964.
15 Cole PV. Nitrous oxide and oxygen from a single cylinder. *Anaesthesia* 1964;**19**:3–11.
16 Tunstall ME. Effect of cooling on pre-mixed gas mixtures for obstetric analgesia. *BMJ* 1963;**ii**:915–17.
17 Cole PV, Crawford JS, Doughty AG *et al.* Specifications and recommendations for nitrous oxide-oxygen apparatus to be used in obstetric analgesia. *Anaesthesia* 1970;**25**:317–27.

18 Doughty, A. The relief of pain in labour: In: Churchill-Davidson HC, ed. *A practice of anaesthesia*, 4th edition. London: Lloyd-Luke (Medical Books) Ltd, 1978:1313.

19 Plantevin OM. *Analgesia and anaesthesia in obstetrics*. London: Butterworths, 1973:75–6.

20 Waud BE, Waud DR. Calculated kinetics of distribution of nitrous oxide and methoxyflurane during intermittent administration in obstetrics. *Anesthesiology* 1970;**32:** 306–16.

21 Mapleson WW. The relation of theoretical pharmacokinetics to clinical anaesthesia. In: Dengler HJ, ed. *Pharmacological and clinical significance of pharmacokinetics*. Stuttgart: Schattauer Verlag, 1969:43–56.

22 McAneny TM, Doughty AG. Self-administered nitrous-oxide/oxygen analgesia in obstetrics. *Anaesthesia* 1963;**18:**488–97.

23 Cole PV, Crawford JS, Doughty AG *et al*. Clinical trials of different concentrations of oxygen and nitrous oxide for obstetric analgesia. Report to the Medical Research Council of the Committee on nitrous oxide and oxygen analgesia in midwifery. *BMJ* 1970;**i:** 709–13.

24 Seward EH. Obstetric analgesia: a new machine for the self-administration of nitrous oxide–oxygen. *Proc R Soc Med* 1949;**42:**745–6.

25 Jones PL, Rosen M, Mushin WW, Jones EV. Methoxyflurane and nitrous oxide as obstetric analgesics. I. A comparison by continuous administration. *BMJ* 1969;**iii:**255–9.

26 Holdcroft A, Morgan M. An assessment of the analgesic effect in labour of pethidine and 50 per cent nitrous oxide in oxygen (Entonox). *J Obstet Gynaecol Br Commonw* 1974;**81:** 603–7.

27 Robinson JO, Rosen M, Evans JM, Revill SI, David H, Rees GAD. Maternal opinion about analgesia for labour. A controlled trial between epidural block and intramuscular pethidine combined with inhalation. *Anaesthesia* 1980;**35:**1173–81.

28 Wraight A. Coping with pain. In: Chamberlain G, Wraight A, Steer P, eds. *Pain and its relief in childbirth: the results of a national survey conducted by the National Birthday Trust*. Edinburgh: Churchill Livingstone, 1993:79–92.

29 Harrison RF, Shore M, Woods T, Mathews G, Gardiner J, Unwin A. A comparative study of transcutaneous electrical nerve stimulation (TENS), entonox, pethidine + promazine and lumbar epidural for pain relief in labor. *Acta Obstet Gynecol Scand* 1987; **66:**9–14.

30 Carstoniu J, Levytam S, Norman P, Daley D, Katz J, Sandler AN. Nitrous oxide in early labor. Safety and analgesic efficacy assessed by a double-blind, placebo-controlled study. *Anesthesiology* 1994;**80:**30–5.

31 Parbrook GD. Therapeutic uses of nitrous oxide: a review. *Br J Anaesth* 1968;**40:**365–72.

32 Willis BA, Rosen M. Entonox analgesia – a method of reducing the delay between demand and supply. *Anaesthesia* 1977;**32:**573–6.

33 Arthurs GJ, Rosen M. Self-administered intermittent nitrous oxide analgesia for labour. Enhancement of effect with continuous nasal inhalation of 50 per cent nitrous oxide (Entonox). *Anaesthesia* 1979;**34:**301–9.

34 Davies JM, Willis BA, Rosen M. Entonox analgesia in labour. A pilot study to reduce the delay between demand and supply. *Anaesthesia* 1978;**33:**545–7.

35 Arthurs GJ, Rosen M. Acceptability of continuous nasal nitrous oxide during labour – a field trial in six maternity hospitals. *Anaesthesia* 1981;**36:**384–8.

36 Levack ID, Tunstall ME. Systems modification in obstetric analgesia. *Anaesthesia* 1984; **39:**183–5.

37 Arora S, Tunstall M, Ross J. Self-administered mixture of Entonox and isoflurane in labour. *Int J Obstet Anesth* 1992;**1:**199–202.

38 Wee MYK, Hasan MA, Thomas TA. Isoflurane in labour. *Anaesthesia* 1993;**48:**369–72.

39 Fadl ET, Utting JE. A study of maternal acid – base state during labour. *Br J Anaesth* 1969;**41:**327–37.

40 Levinson G, Shnider SM, DeLorimier AA, Steffenson JL. Effects of maternal hyperventilation on uterine blood flow and fetal oxygenation and acid–base status. *Anesthesiology* 1974;**40:**340–7.

41 Motoyama EK, Rivard G, Acheson F, Cook CD. Adverse effect of maternal hyperventilation on the foetus. *Lancet* 1966;**i:**286–8.

42 Reed PN, Colquhoun AD, Hanning CD. Maternal oxygenation during normal labour. *Br J Anaesth* 1989;**62:**316–18.

43 Griffin RP, Reynolds F. Maternal hypoxaemia during labour and delivery: the influence of analgesia and effect on neonatal outcome. *Anaesthesia* 1995;**50:**151–6.

44 Huch A, Huch R, Schneider H, Rooth G. Continuous transcutaneous monitoring of fetal oxygen tension during labour. *Br J Obstet Gynaecol* 1977;**84**(Suppl. 1):1–39.

45 Prowse CM, Gaensler EA. Respiratory and acid–base changes during pregnancy. *Anesthesiology* 1965;**26:**381–92.

46 Lin DM, Reisner LS, Benumof J. Hypoxemia occurs intermittently and significantly with nitrous oxide labor analgesia. *Anesth Analg* 1989;**68:**S167.

47 Deckardt R, Fembacher PM, Schneider KTM, Graeff H. Maternal arterial oxygen saturation during labor and delivery: pain-dependent alterations and effects on the newborn. *Obstet Gynecol* 1987;**70:**21–5.

48 Zelcer J, Owers H, Paull JD. A controlled oximetric evaluation of inhalational, opioid and epidural analgesia in labour. *Anaesth Intens Care* 1989;**17:**418–21

49 Davies JM, Hogg M, Rosen M. Maternal arterial oxygen tension during intermittent inhalation analgesia. *Br J Anaesth* 1975;**47:**370–8.

50 Wilkins CJ, Reed PN, Aitkenhead AR. Hypoxaemia after inhalation of 50% nitrous oxide and oxygen. *Br J Anaesth* 1989;**63:**346–7.

51 Amos RJ, Amess JAL, Hinds CJ, Mollin DL. Incidence and pathogenesis of acute megaloblastic bone-marrow change in patients receiving intensive care. *Lancet* 1982;**ii:** 835–8.

52 Amess JAL, Burman JF, Rees GM, Nancekievill DG, Mollin DL. Megaloblastic haemopoiesis in patients receiving nitrous oxide. *Lancet* 1978;**ii:**339–42.

53 Layzer RB. Myeloneuropathy after prolonged exposure to nitrous oxide. *Lancet* 1978;**ii:** 1227–30.

54 Jacobson B, Nyberg K, Eklund G, Bygdeman M, Rydberg U. Obstetric pain medication and eventual adult amphetamine addiction in offspring. *Acta Obstet Gynecol Scand* 1988; **67:**677–82.

55 Jacobson B, Nyberg K, Grönbladh L, Eklund G, Bygdeman M, Rydberg U. Opiate addiction in adult offspring through possible imprinting after obstetric treatment. *BMJ* 1990;**301:**1067–70.

56 Crawford JS, Tunstall ME. Notes on respiratory performance during labour. *Br J Anaesth* 1968;**40:**612–14.

57 Moir DD. *Obstetric Anaesthesia and Analgesia.* London, Baillière Tindall, 1976:53.

58 Stefani SJ, Hughes SC, Shnider SM, *et al.* Neonatal neurobehavioral effects of inhalational analgesia for vaginal delivery. *Anesthesiology* 1982;**56:**351–5.

59 Hay DM. Nitrous oxide transfer across the placenta and condition of the newborn at delivery. *Br J Obstet Gynaecol* 1978;**85:**299–302.

60 Gamsu H. The effects of pain relief on the baby. In: Chamberlain G, Wraight A, Steer P, eds. *Pain and its relief in childbirth: the results of a national survey conducted by the National Birthday Trust.* Edinburgh: Churchill Livingstone, 1993:93–100.

61 Moir DD. *Obstetric Anaesthesia and Analgesia.* London, Baillière Tindall, 1976:107.

62 Phillips TJ, Macdonald RR. Comparative effect of pethidine, trichloroethylene, and Entonox on fetal and neonatal acid-base and Po_2. *BMJ* 1971;**iii:**558–60.

63 Crandell WB, Macdonald A. Nephropathy associated with methoxyflurane anesthesia. A follow-up report. *JAMA* 1968;**205:**798–9.

64 Frascino JA, Vanamee P, Rosen PP. Renal oxalosis and azotemia after methoxyflurane anesthesia. *N Engl J Med* 1970;**283:**676–9.

65 Crandell WB, Pappas SG, Macdonald A. Nephrotoxicity associated with methoxyflurane anesthesia. *Anesthesiology* 1966;**27:**591–607.

66 Lebowitz MH. Nephrogenic diabetes insipidus following methoxyflurane anesthesia. A report of two cases. *Anesth Analg* 1969;**48:**233–6.

67 Merkle RB, McDonald FD, Waldman J *et al.* Human renal function following methoxyflurane anesthesia. *JAMA* 1971;**218:**841–4.

68 Panner BJ, Freeman RB, Roth-Moyo LA, Markowitch W. Toxicity following methoxyflurane anesthesia. *JAMA* 1970;**214:**86–90.

69 Pezzi PJ, Frobese AS, Greenberg SR. Methoxyflurane and renal toxicity. *Lancet* 1966;**i:** 823.
70 Cousins MJ, Mazze RI. Methoxyflurane nephrotoxicity. A study of dose response in man. *JAMA* 1973;**225:**1611–16.
71 Creasser CW, Stoelting RK, Krishna G, Peterson C. Methoxyflurane metabolism and renal function after methoxyflurane analgesia during labor and delivery. *Anesthesiology* 1974;**41:**62–6.
72 Rubinger D, Davidson JT, Melmed RN. Hepatitis following the use of methoxyflurane in obstetric analgesia. *Anesthesiology* 1975;**43:**593–5.
73 Clark RB, Cooper JO, Brown WE, Greifenstein FE. The effect of methoxyflurane on the foetus. *Br J Anaesth* 1970;**42:**286–94.
74 Chase RE, Holaday DA, Fiserova-Bergerova V, Saidman LJ, Mack FE. The biotransformation of Ethrane in man. *Anesthesiology* 1971;**35:**262–7.
75 Holaday DA, Fiserova-Bergerova V, Latto IP, Zumbiel MA. Resistance of isoflurane to biotransformation in man. *Anesthesiology* 1975;**43:**325–32.
76 Mazze RI, Calverley RK, Smith NT. Inorganic fluoride nephrotoxicity: prolonged enflurane and halothane anesthesia in volunteers. *Anesthesiology* 1977;**46:**265–71.
77 Dobkin AB, Kim D, Choi JK, Levy AA. Blood serum fluoride levels with enflurane (Ethrane) and isoflurane (Forane) anaesthesia during and following major abdominal surgery. *Can Anaesth Soc J* 1973;**20:**494–8.
78 McGuinness C, Rosen M. Enflurane as an analgesic in labour. *Anaesthesia* 1984;**39:**24–6.
79 McLeod DD, Ramayya GP, Tunstall ME. Self-administered isoflurane in labour. A comparative study with Entonox. *Anaesthesia* 1985;**40:**424–6.
80 Tunstall ME, Ross JAS. Isoflurane, nitrous oxide and oxygen analgesic mixtures [Letter]. *Anaesthesia* 1993;**48:**919.
81 Cousins MJ, Greenstein LR, Hitt BA, Mazze RI. Metabolism and renal effects of enflurane in man. *Anesthesiology* 1976;**44:**44–53.
82 Buring JE, Hennekens CH, Mayrent SL, Rosner B, Greenberg ER, Colton T. Health experiences of operating room personnel. *Anesthesiology* 1985;**62:**325–30.
83 Vieira E, Cleaton-Jones P, Moyes D. Effects of low intermittent concentrations of nitrous oxide on the developing rat fetus. *Br J Anaesth* 1983;**55:**67–9.
84 Lane GA, Nahrwold ML, Tait AR, Taylor-Busch M, Cohen PJ, Beaudoin AR. Anesthetics as teratogens: nitrous oxide is fetotoxic, xenon is not. *Science* 1980;**210:**899–901.
85 Corbett TH, Cornell RG, Endres JL, Millard RI. Effects of low concentrations of nitrous oxide on rat pregnancy. *Anesthesiology* 1973;**39:**299–301.
86 Vieira E, Cleaton-Jones P, Austin JC, Moyes DG, Shaw R. Effects of low concentrations of nitrous oxide on rat fetuses. *Anesth Analg* 1980;**59:**175–7.
87 Cohen EN, Bellville JW, Brown BW. Anesthesia, pregnancy, and miscarriage: a study of operating room nurses and anesthetists. *Anesthesiology* 1971;**35:**343–7.
88 Spence AA. Environmental pollution by inhalation anaesthetics. *Br J Anaesth* 1987;**59:** 96–103.
89 Halsey MJ. *Anaesthesia rounds. Occupational exposure to inhalational anaesthetics.* Oxford: The Medicine Group (Education) Ltd, 1996:5.
90 Health and Safety Executive. EH40/96. *Occupational exposure limits.* London: HMSO, 1996.
91 Davenport HT, Halsey MJ, Wardley-Smith B, Bateman PE. Occupational exposure to anaesthetics in 20 hospitals. *Anaesthesia* 1980;**35:**354–9.
92 Sweeney B, Bingham RM, Amos RJ, Petty AC, Cole PV. Toxicity of bone marrow in dentists exposed to nitrous oxide. *BMJ* 1985;**291:**567–9.
93 Hillman KM, Saloojee Y, Brett II, Cole PV. Nitrous oxide concentrations in the dental surgery. *Anaesthesia* 1981;**36:**257–62.
94 Mills GH, Singh D, Longan M, O'Sullivan J, Caunt JA. Nitrous oxide exposure on the labour ward. *Int J Obstet Anesth* 1996;**5:**160–4.

5: Systemic opioid analgesia

Introduction

Opioids have been used for analgesia in labour for hundreds of years, often as an incidental component of a complex potion. The Greeks and Romans used opium, which in some cases was mixed with mandragora, an extract from the mandragon plant containing hyoscine.[1] Historical texts from the sixteenth and seventeenth centuries report the use of many elaborate herbal concoctions, used topically or taken orally, many of which contained opioids.[2] However, it was not until the early twentieth century that techniques deliberately employing the analgesic effects of the opioids gained major attention.

Around this time twilight sleep, a combination of morphine and hyoscine, started to gain popularity – albeit more among the pregnant mothers than their medical attendants.[3] The technique, developed in Germany and first described in 1902, involved giving a single dose of morphine followed by intermittent doses of hyoscine titrated according to the individual mother's "needs". As with most systemic opioids, before and since, the quality of analgesia was poor. However the women became sedated and, in about 95% of cases, had no recollection of the experience of labour and childbirth. The amnesic effect was the cause of its widespread popularity but because of its obvious dangers, twilight sleep could only be administered in the hospital setting, and this led to a campaign for more hospital admissions among its enthusiasts. In its early years, physicians would titrate the dose to each mother individually, limiting its availability. Later, attempts were made to standardise the technique and broaden its application. However the side effects were severe. Hyoscine caused hallucinations and delirium often necessitating physical restraint. This delirium was reduced by nursing the woman in a quiet, darkened room, making it more difficult to monitor her. The newborn baby was removed quickly so that its cries did not disturb her, although often the neonatal depression caused by the technique made this unnecessary. These dangers led to its growing unpopularity within the medical profession, but it took considerable maternal and neonatal mortality and morbidity to convince its proponents likewise. Some attempts were made to improve the cocktail by adding barbiturates but generally such changes only increased the dangers and the technique was largely abandoned by the end of the 1930s.

The 1930s heralded the introduction of pethidine which has since become the most commonly used and widely investigated systemic opioid in labour.[4] Pethidine was developed in Germany during the First World War as a substitute for morphine, which was unavailable in Germany due to an Allied embargo. Pethidine was promoted for its analgesic and spasmolytic properties and made freely available. It became very popular among midwives and labouring women, many of whom, unaware of its addictive properties, became dependent on the drug. It was not until the Dangerous Drugs Act of 1949 that its use became restricted.

Currently possession and administration of pethidine by midwives is regulated under the Medicines Act 1968 and the Misuse of Drugs Regulations 1985,[5] although it was made legally available to midwives in 1950. It is this availability and ease of administration that has resulted in the continued widespread use of systemic opioids in labour despite overwhelming evidence of their lack of efficacy and their detrimental effects on both mother and baby.

General pharmacology

An opiate is defined as a drug that is derived from opium, which itself is an extract of the poppy, *Papaver somniferum*. Such drugs include morphine, codeine, thebaine and substances derived directly from them. An opioid is defined as any drug that has agonist and/or antagonist activity at an opioid receptor and embraces the naturally occurring opioid peptides and synthetic opioid bases.

Opioid receptors

Although suspected for many years, the first conclusive evidence that several different subtypes of opioid receptors existed came from studies demonstrating "cross-tolerance" among opioids in animal experiments. Martin *et al* demonstrated the existence of three receptor subtypes, μ, κ and σ, named after the drugs that bound to them, morphine, ketocyclazocine and SKF 10 047 (N-allylnormetazocine).[6] The σ receptor is no longer considered a true opioid receptor as it has no affinity for the opioid antagonist naloxone. However, in 1977 Lord *et al* proposed the existence of a fourth receptor, δ.[7] Opioid receptors are widely acknowledged to be coupled to guanine nucleotide G proteins.[8] Activation of opioid receptors causes inhibition of neural transmission either by potassium channel activation that results in hyperpolarisation (μ and δ) or by inhibition of voltage-dependent calcium channels (κ and δ).[9,10]

More recently, the three accepted opioid receptor subtypes have been further divided and it is likely that more will be identified in future. μ receptors have been subdivided into two groups: μ_1 receptors are present predominantly in the brain and mediate analgesia and sedation centrally, μ_2 receptors mediate analgesia in the dorsal column of the spinal cord. Other μ_2 receptors are thought to be responsible for respiratory depression and for decreasing motility in the gastrointestinal tract.[11] Though growing numbers of new receptor subtypes are being identified, and debate continues concerning their physiological roles, only the simplest classification is required for a general understanding of opioid behaviour (Table 5.1).

Agonists, partial agonists, and antagonists

Drugs that bind to opioid receptors are grouped into three categories: agonists, partial agonists and antagonists (Table 5.2). Drugs such as morphine and fentanyl are agonists because they bind to opioid receptors and, in large doses, cause profound analgesia. Other drugs such as buprenorphine and pentazocine are incapable of producing profound analgesia at high doses having a low maximum effect. These drugs have a lower efficacy than morphine, fentanyl and pethidine and are partial

TABLE 5.1—*Opioid receptor function*

Receptor	Function
μ	Analgesia to thermal and chemical stimuli
	Central analgesia (μ_1)
	Spinal analgesia (μ_2)
	Euphoria and dependence
	Gastrointestinal effects
	Respiratory depression
	Pruritus
κ	Analgesia to chemical stimuli
	Spinal analgesia
	Sedation
δ	Analgesia to thermal stimuli
	? Gastrointestinal effects
	? Respiratory depression
σ*	Dysphoria

*No longer classified as a true opioid receptor.
Based on Reynolds[12]

TABLE 5.2—*Actions of opioid drugs at different receptors*

	Receptor	
Drug	μ	κ
Pethidine	+ +	+
Morphine	+ + +	+
Meptazinol	+/−	+
Pentazocine	+/−	+
Nalbuphine	−	+
Fentanyl	+ + +	
Buprenorphine	+/−	−
Naloxone	− −	−

+ Agonist; +/− Partial agonist; − Antagonist.

agonists. Some partial agonists have a very high affinity for opioid receptors despite low efficacy and may therefore act as antagonists by displacing molecules of higher efficacy but lower affinity from receptors. For example, buprenorphine displaces morphine from the μ receptor thereby antagonising its analgesic effect. κ receptors are unable to mediate as profound analgesia as μ receptors. Hence opioids that bind principally to κ receptors may appear to be partial agonists because they have low maximum effects. Pure antagonists such as naloxone bind with high affinity to opioid receptors but have no efficacy.

Physicochemical properties

Physicochemical properties of opioids (Table 5.3) have important bearings on their disposition and fate in the body. High lipid solubility enhances

TABLE 5.3—*Physicochemical and pharmacological properties of opioids*

Opioid	Molecular weight	Apparent oil-buffer partition coefficient			Protein binding (%)	Half-life (h)
		Octanol	Oleyl alcohol	Heptane		
Pethidine	247	39	18		30–65	3–5
Morphine	285	1·4			30	1·4–4
Nalbuphine	357				34	2·4
Meptazinol	234				30	2
Fentanyl	336	77	550	9	84	8
Buprenorphine	467			2000	96	2–5

Adapted from Reynolds[12]

speed of onset and increases the volume of distribution. Hence, after bolus i.v. injection, drug is initially rapidly cleared from the circulation, though the terminal half-life may be prolonged. The opioids in common use have molecular weights between 200 and 500 (Table 5.3). They all contain a basic nitrogen, usually in the form of a piperidine group (Figure 5.1). These groups can accept a proton in acid solution thereby becoming ionised and hydrophilic. However it is the non-ionised moiety that is able to cross lipid membranes most rapidly. Morphine possesses two hydroxyl groups (Figure 5.1) that reduce the lipophilicity of the molecule and slow the rate at which it crosses lipid membranes.[13] In the related molecule diacetyl

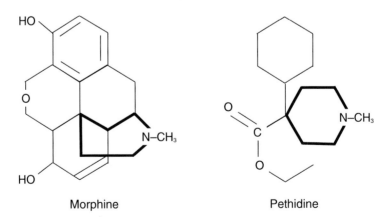

Morphine   Pethidine

FIGURE 5.1—*The structural formulae of morphine and pethidine. The piperidine ring in each is highlighted.*

morphine (diamorphine), these groups are substituted with more lipophilic acetyl groups allowing rapid passage of the molecule across the blood–brain barrier and faster onset of action. Pethidine and other phenylpiperidine derivatives such as fentanyl and sufentanil are also more lipid-soluble than morphine and have more rapid onset of action (Table 5.3).

Protein binding

Hydrophobic drugs tend to be highly protein-bound in the plasma. Most opioids, like many basic drugs, are principally bound to the acute phase protein α_1-acid glycoprotein. This is of particular relevance in obstetric analgesia, as while albumin concentrations are higher in fetus than mother, maternal levels of α_1-acid glycoprotein are higher than fetal,[14] and this to some degree reduces placental transfer of the drug to the fetus, though not enough to prevent the neonatal side effects discussed later. One important exception is fentanyl which is bound to several protein fractions including albumin; binding may therefore be as great in fetus as in mother, representing a larger burden of drug to the newborn. This bound moiety may, moreover, become unbound in the neonatal period.

Fate

Morphine is conjugated in the liver to produce morphine-3-glucuronide and, to a lesser extent, morphine-6-glucuronide, both of which are excreted in the urine. Morphine-6-glucuronide has analgesic activity and may accumulate in renal failure. Pethidine is first dealkylated in the liver to produce its principal metabolite, norpethidine. Both molecules are then hydrolysed, conjugated and eliminated in the urine. Norpethidine produces analgesia, sedation, is proconvulsant and has a prolonged half-life in both mother (17–25 h) and neonate (62 h).[15]

Mode of action

Opioids produce analgesia by actions in at least four primary sites: the peri-aqueductal grey matter, the nucleus raphe magnus, the locus ceruleus and the dorsal horn of the spinal cord, principally in the superficial layers of the spinal grey matter, laminae I, II and III (Figure 5.2).

Stimulation of opioid receptors in the peri-aqueductal grey matter activates descending inhibitory pathways passing via the nucleus raphe magnus to be relayed down to the dorsal horn cells. This results in serotoninergic inhibition of the dorsal horn relay neurones leading to analgesia. Other descending pathways activated by opioid binding within

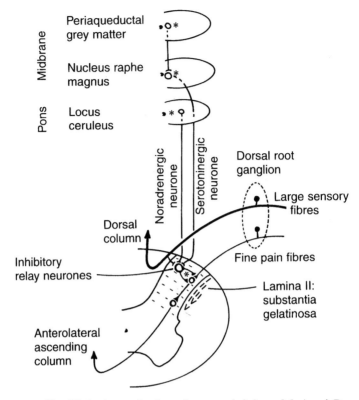

FIGURE 5.2—*Simplified scheme of pain pathways and their modulation. * Denotes sites where opiate receptors are found. Pain transmission is inhibited by collaterals from large sensory fibres, descending inhibitory fibres and opiate agonists acting on receptors in the dorsal horn.*

the locus ceruleus result in noradrenergic inhibition at the dorsal horn. Interruption of the descending pathways has been shown to attenuate the analgesic response to systemic opioids.[16] In the dorsal horn itself there are opioid receptors on the relay neurones that inhibit the transmission of nocioceptive stimuli.

Systemic opioids given to provide analgesia in labour act primarily within the central nervous system at a supra-spinal level. The increased lipid solubility of pethidine compared to morphine fueled the hope that it would provide superior analgesia because it could reach its site of action more quickly. Unfortunately, as with all systemic opioids, the dose of pethidine required to produce adequate analgesia in labour by this mechanism results in unacceptable sedation and respiratory depression in both mother and newborn. Administration of opioids by the spinal root greatly enhances their analgesic effect.[17]

Pethidine, having very low potency, is given in such a high dose that it has a direct membrane stabilising action similar to that of a local anaesthetic.[18] Although this property cannot contribute to the effect of systemically administered pethidine, it contributes to its effect on epidural or spinal application. Similar properties have not been demonstrated with other opioids because they are given at lower doses.

Pethidine (meperidine)

Of the opioids, pethidine is the most widely used in labour in the UK (Table 5.4) and has been the most extensively studied both here and in the USA.

TABLE 5.4—*Frequency and type of opioid analgesia used in the UK*

Opioid receptor agonists	Availability (%)	Maternal usage* (%)
Pethidine (meperidine)	97·6	36·9/37·8
Diamorphine	<5	2·1/3·6
Meptazinol (meptid)	<5	1·8/3·3

*Midwife reported/maternal reported.

Based on National Birthday Trust survey[19]

Efficacy

Despite many anecdotal reports and a number of retrospective trials suggesting that pethidine provides satisfactory analgesia, the overwhelming majority of prospective trials continue to report that pethidine is, at best, a poor analgesic in labour.

A fundamental problem with many studies that describe good analgesic results from pethidine is the manner in which pain assessment was made. Independent observers commonly report good analgesic effect based on the fact that the parturient appears calmer and quieter following injection of pethidine.[20] Direct questioning of labouring women reveals that though they may feel more sleepy, there has been little or no improvement in pain.[21,22] Thus sedation, which is potentially harmful for the mother and may detract from her experience of birth, has become confused with analgesia. Similarly it has been shown that mothers asked to score their labour pain retrospectively 24 hours after delivery report significantly less

93

pain than they did during labour.[23] Accurate assessment of pain during labour and effect of analgesic intervention can only, therefore, be made by the parturient at the time of labour.

In the step-ladder of obstetric analgesia there is a general belief among childbirth educators and mothers that harmless, non-invasive techniques come first (psychological preparation and support, massage, warm baths, TENS etc.), followed by nitrous oxide and then finally, if stronger analgesia is required, pethidine or epidural. Although non-invasive techniques are well qualified for the lower part of the ladder, much research suggests that, in reality, pethidine hardly reaches the bottom rung. In their study of 663 labouring mothers, Holdcroft and Morgan showed that nitrous oxide produced satisfactory analgesia in almost 50% whereas pethidine failed to do so in over 75%.[24] In another study a combination of pethidine and promazine was shown to provide inferior analgesia to TENS; 96% of the TENS group compared to only 54% of the pethidine + promazine reported partial pain relief although in both groups approximately 80% required further analgesia. In the same study, 90% of patients who received nitrous oxide reported partial pain relief, and only one in twenty required further analgesia.[25]

A number of studies have shown that pain scores may actually increase after pethidine analgesia (see Figure 3.3).[26,27] In both cases this increase in pain scores was put down to the progress of labour. A more recent study comparing the effect of pethidine and morphine on pain scores during labour showed no significant change in pain over time or between the groups while at the same time demonstrating no change in the intensity of labour as measured by an intrauterine pressure transducer (Figure 5.3).[22]

Pethidine has, in recent years, been compared with several other systemic opioids. On each occasion it was hoped that the alternatives would supply superior analgesia with improved side effect profiles. However, in the vast majority of cases, analgesia was similar and side effects little altered. These comparisons will be discussed under the individual drugs (see below). Pethidine has also been compared with intramuscular injections of ketorolac. Although ketorolac produced fewer maternal and neonatal side effects, analgesia was inferior.[28] It is unlikely that non-steroidal anti-inflammatory drugs will gain popularity for analgesia in labour because of the perceived risk of adverse effects on the fetal circulation – in particular vasoconstriction and premature closure of the ductus arteriosus.

Finally, systemic pethidine has been compared with epidural analgesia in a few randomised trials, which of course demonstrated clinically inferior analgesia.[27,29,30]

There have been a number of attempts to improve the efficacy of pethidine by administering it in combination with other drugs. In general

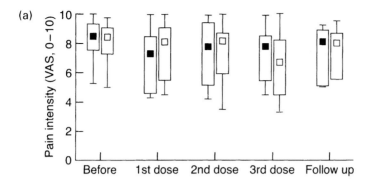

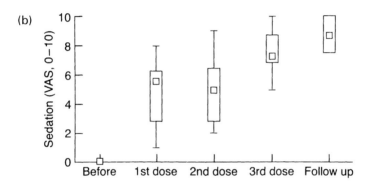

FIGURE 5.3—(a) Pain intensity and (b) sedation scores, before and after morphine 0.05 mg/kg (filled squares) or pethidine 0.5 mg/kg (open squares) up to 3 doses given intravenously every 3 contractions to parturients. Boxes represent median and interquartile ranges, and whiskers total range. Sedation scores in the two groups have been combined. Follow up = 30 min later. (From Olofsson et al[22] by permission of the authors and publisher)

such combinations have only increased sedation, amnesia and dysphoria while having little impact on analgesia.[31] There is some suggestion that the addition of the antiemetic metoclopramide may improve analgesia, though evidence is inconsistent.[32–34] It has been recognised for a number of years that the addition of promethazine to opioids has an anti-analgesic effect and this has been borne out in labour.[34]

Other attempts to improve the efficacy of pethidine have involved using different routes and modes of delivery (see below).

There are unfortunately no randomised trials to compare pethidine with placebo. In the past such trials have been considered unethical. However, the evidence that we now have suggests that the analgesic efficacy of pethidine is little better than that of a placebo while the side effects are considerably more serious. Thus, such a trial would no longer be unethical.

Effects on the mother

Central nervous system

In the national survey of pain relief in childbirth sponsored by the National Birthday Trust, pethidine received wide-ranging criticism from the mothers who used it.[19] In particular they complained of feelings of confusion, loss of control and feeling sleepy in the face of minimal, if any, pain relief. A few found pethidine helpful although in the majority of these cases they admitted that this was not because it reduced their pain but more because it made them less concerned about it. Sedation is consistently a prominent feature in systemic pethidine administration.

Gastrointestinal tract

Perhaps more important is the effect that pethidine has on maternal gastrointestinal function. Although nausea and vomiting are common in labour, the administration of pethidine has been shown to increase the incidence of these complications (Figure 5.4).

An antiemetic such as metoclopramide or prochlorperazine reduces these side effects and should always be given with pethidine. Metoclopramide

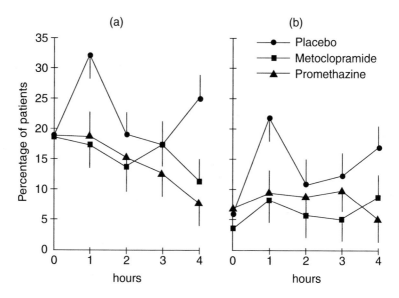

FIGURE 5.4—*Percentage of patients with (a) nausea and (b) vomiting, before (time 0) and in the four hours after intramuscular pethidine with placebo, metoclopramide or promethazine. Vertical bars represent standard errors of the proportions. Significantly more patients in the placebo group had nausea and vomiting. (Modified from Vella et al*[34] *by permission of the publisher)*

may be the antiemetic of choice since it promotes gastric emptying and does not cause sedation. Nimmo *et al* clearly demonstrated using a paracetamol absorption technique that parenteral opioid analgesics delayed gastric emptying.[35] Holdsworth *et al*, studying women who progressed to caesarean section under general anaesthesia, demonstrated that administration of pethidine in labour greatly increased the residual gastric volumes, up to 700 ml in one individual.[36] Although administration of metoclopramide may mitigate against this somewhat, it cannot be guaranteed to eliminate the danger.[37] A parturient who has been given pethidine might be considered more likely to require general anaesthesia in the event of an emergency caesarean section because she either could not or would not have regional anaesthesia in labour. Such a parturient is at increased risk of aspiration because of the combination of greater residual gastric volume and the physiological changes in pregnancy that promote gastro-oesophageal reflux.[38]

In this era of changing childbirth one of the changes being enthusiastically advocated by many midwives, obstetricians and some anaesthetists is the liberalisation of eating policies for labouring women.[39] The administration of pethidine must surely be a contraindication to oral intake in labour (see Chapter 6). Furthermore:

parturients receiving pethidine should automatically receive both ranitidine and metoclopramide at the same time.

Respiratory system

Despite the age-old belief that pain is a normal, physiological and perhaps even beneficial accompaniment to labour, there is some evidence that it may be of some detriment above and beyond the psychological trauma it metes upon some mothers. Severe pain and distress cause labouring mothers to hyperventilate during contractions. This has potentially harmful sequelae. During a contraction, hyperventilation causes the maternal arterial carbon dioxide tension ($Paco_2$) to fall, resulting in a degree of maternal vasoconstriction which may compromise uterine artery blood flow and, possibly more importantly, increases maternal haemoglobin affinity for oxygen.[40] Between contractions the reduced maternal $Paco_2$ combined with exhaustion may result in hypoxic episodes due to underventilation or periods of apnoea.[40,41] The administration of pethidine exacerbates this problem as it provides minimal reduction of the pain and hyperventilation during contraction, and yet causes a degree of sedation between contractions that exacerbates the periods of underventilation and apnoea.[42]

Effect on the progress of labour

Several theories have been put forward over the years concerning the effect of opioids in general and pethidine in particular on the progress of labour.

97

Before the 1960s it was generally felt that all forms of analgesia, conduction anaesthesia and opioids alike, slowed the progress of labour.[43] The mechanism of this effect was never clarified, nor was it established by randomised trial, although more recently opioids have been shown experimentally to reduce maternal and fetal oxytocin levels, providing a possible explanation. In animal studies morphine and pethidine have both been shown to reduce oxytocin production and to delay parturition.[44,45] Lindow et al demonstrated a similar reduction in plasma oxytocin levels in the first stage of labour following intravenous morphine in humans, though this effect has yet to be demonstrated with pethidine.[46] It is unclear whether doses used in labour of either drug would be sufficient to affect the progress of labour.[47] Thornton et al showed that the administration of pethidine caused no change in fetal oxytocin production whereas epidural analgesia appeared to increase it.[48] Though it had been suggested that fetal oxytocin may influence the onset and duration of labour, high levels of cystine aminopeptidase, an enzyme that rapidly degrades oxytocin in the placenta, mitigates against significant feto-maternal transfer.[49]

It has also been suggested that rather than slowing labour, pethidine may actually accelerate it. Furthermore, it is not an uncommon view among midwives that pethidine is the analgesic of choice in early labour for this very reason. Though the effect itself has not been established, a number of rather tenuous explanations for it have been proposed. Pajntar et al demonstrated that pethidine given in the active phase of labour was associated with an increase in contractility of the body of the uterus but a concomitant decrease in the contractility of the cervix.[50] They suggested that this explained how pethidine might accelerate the progress of labour by facilitating cervical dilatation. However, the changes they noted did not correlate with the duration of the active phase of labour. A second suggestion was put forward by Milwidsky et al who demonstrated that pethidine in therapeutic concentration stimulates urokinase, plasmin and collagenase activity in vitro.[51] They proposed that these enzymes were responsible for degrading cervical collagen and elastin leading to accelerated cervical effacement and dilatation during labour.

There remains, however, no clinical trial demonstrating that pethidine shortens either the active or passive phases of labour.

Effects on the baby

The effects of pethidine on the baby depend on the combination of its physical properties, which dictate the rate and extent of its transfer to the fetus across the placenta, and its pharmacological actions, including those of its active metabolite, norpethidine.

Pethidine is a weakly basic piperidine derivative which possesses about one-third the lipophilicity of methadone and one-thirtieth that of fentanyl, though it is 20–30 times more lipophilic than morphine (see Table 5.3). This degree of lipophilicity allows pethidine to diffuse rapidly across the placenta such that it can theoretically approach transplacental equilibrium in a single circuit, although equilibrium deeper into the fetal compartment may take considerably longer. Thus, rate of diffusion is not limited by permeability but is dependent on the rate at which it is delivered to the placenta and removed into the fetus (flow-dependant transfer). Morphine, which is less lipophilic, diffuses more slowly across the placental membrane and its transfer is therefore partially limited by permeability.[52]

Two further factors influencing transplacental passage of pethidine are protein binding and degree of ionisation. Pethidine is principally bound to α_1-acid glycoprotein (30–60%). At term levels of this protein tend to be higher in maternal than fetal circulation and in theory therefore to favour distribution of pethidine more into maternal than fetal compartment. However, this relatively weak binding appears to have little effect in practice.[53] On the other hand, pH gradients across the placenta may be of greater importance. As a weak base, pethidine is ionised to a greater extent in the more acidic milieu of the fetal circulation. Thus, a certain degree of ion trapping may occur on the fetal side of the placenta increasing fetal uptake of the drug. In the normal situation, the pH of the fetal circulation is only slightly more acidic than that of the mother and therefore the disparity in concentration of free drug is not great. However, in the compromised fetus, acidosis may increase and the ion trapping effect may become exaggerated, resulting in increased fetal concentrations of pethidine and concomitant side effects.[54]

The neonatal side effects of pethidine, respiratory depression in particular, have been shown to be most severe if the dose delivery interval is 2–3 hours.[55,56] It has been suggested that this is due to gradual distribution of pethidine and norpethidine into the fetal compartment, plus fetal conversion of pethidine to norpethidine, that leads to persistent transplacental passage of pethidine into the fetus for some time after maternal plasma concentrations have started to fall. This continuous increase of total fetal dose of pethidine, together with a progressive rise in fetal norpethidine concentration, can result in long-lasting neonatal depression and is of course augmented by repeated maternal dosing which traditionally occurs 3–4 hourly.[15]

The neonatal side effects of pethidine are compounded by the production of its active metabolite norpethidine. Originally it was believed that both the mother and baby were unable to metabolise pethidine to norpethidine.[57] However, there is now little doubt that they both do and that, in the baby, most of the norpethidine probably results from its own N-dealkylation.[58-60]

Norpethidine does have analgesic activity, though it is considerably less potent than pethidine. However, it causes more respiratory depression and has pro-convulsant properties.[56,61] The half-lives of pethidine and norpethidine in the mother are approximately 4 and 20 hours respectively but in the neonate these are 13 and 62 hours.[15,58] These prolonged half-lives probably explain why many of the behavioural changes observed in exposed neonates persist for several days after delivery.

Effects of pethidine on the fetus

A number of studies have demonstrated fetal changes occurring within minutes of administration of intramuscular pethidine to the mother. Changes have been observed in fetal heart rate pattern (reduced variability),[62,63] fetal breathing movements and muscular activity,[64] fetal EEG activity[65] and fetal scalp oxygen tension.[66] The bearing that these changes may have on fetal well-being is unclear, but it is possible that changes in heart rate may result in unnecessary intervention. Thalme et al reported impaired fetal acid–base balance following maternal administration of small doses of pethidine (compared to epidural babies), and these changes persisted after delivery.[67] However, what may be more important are the effects that are apparent at birth, principally respiratory depression and behavioural changes.

Early neonatal effects

Neonatal respiratory depression caused by maternal administration of pethidine is extensively documented and, as explained previously, is worst after a dose delivery interval of about three hours and particularly after repeated maternal doses.[15,55,56] This respiratory depression results in decreased Apgar scores, depressed oxygen saturations and increased arterial carbon dioxide tensions.[55,68,69]

Even in the absence of clinically obvious respiratory depression at the time of birth, a number of groups have reported more subtle changes in respiratory patterns in the first few days of life. Hamza et al studied a group of babies whose mothers had received infusions of pethidine in labour. When compared with a control opioid-free group, Apgar scores were not depressed and in quiet sleep the groups were indistinguishable. However, in active sleep Sao_2 levels <90% and apnoeic episodes were more common in the pethidine group.[70]

There are many studies of neurobehavioural changes following delivery in babies exposed to pethidine in utero. The multitude of factors that affect early neonatal behaviour make such studies difficult to control. Furthermore, the difficulties in design and interpretation of the various neonatal behavioural scoring systems leave many of these studies open to criticism. Several studies have suggested that such babies are sleepy, less able to develop suckling skills and therefore take longer to establish breast feeding.[71–73] This, combined with the observation by Bernard *et al* that large doses of pethidine given to mothers result in impaired thermoregulation in the newborn, may increase the need for medical intervention in the early hours of life.[74]

The effects of pethidine on the baby can be rapidly reversed immediately after delivery with an adequate dose of intramuscular naloxone, an opioid antagonist. Although naloxone has a slightly prolonged half-life in the newborn, it is shorter than that of pethidine (3 hours compared with 20 hours approximately), and therefore needs to be given intramuscularly in a large dose to have a sufficiently prolonged effect.[75] Naloxone is, moreover, less able to antagonise the effects of the longer-acting norpethidine than those of pethidine. An appropriate dose of naloxone in the newborn is 60–100 µg/kg which appears to have a clinical effect for up to 48 hours and reverses the neurobehavioural effects of pethidine without apparent harm to the newborn.[76,77] If opioid effects are marked, respiratory support with bag and face mask or even intubation and ventilation may be required in addition to naloxone, particularly when the narcotic effect of pethidine is superimposed on any other cause of fetal compromise. However, in babies of sickle cell patients or chronic drug abusers, who have been exposed in utero for a prolonged period to excessive doses of pethidine or other opioids, naloxone may cause severe withdrawal reactions including convulsions and coma and should therefore be avoided.

Late effects

Some evidence has emerged that babies of mothers who received pethidine during labour might be more liable to develop drug addiction problems later in life. Jacobson *et al* compared the intrapartum care of mothers of 200 opioid addicts with that of unaffected siblings. They showed that the mother was more likely to have had pethidine during labour in the addict group. Although the control group was poorly matched – it contained a larger proportion of girls – and the study was retrospective, it does raise the possibility of a particularly disturbing long-term side effect of a drug that remains in such widespread use.[78]

Contraindications and drug interactions

All systemic opioid drugs licensed for use in labour have some degree of sedative action. As a result they potentiate sedation caused by any other drug that the parturient may have been given (e.g. benzodiazepines, anti-epileptic drugs, magnesium sulphate and some antidepressants). Furthermore, if large doses of opioids have been given in labour, subsequent removal of stimuli by effective regional analgesia may result in heavy

101

maternal sedation. Indeed respiratory arrest has been reported in such circumstances.[79]

Pethidine is absolutely contraindicated in any parturient who is taking *monoamine oxidase inhibitors* as it may precipitate a sympathomimetic crisis. Although these drugs are now rarely prescribed because of their dangerous side effects, they are not specifically contraindicated in pregnancy. Ironically, the fact that they are now so little used means that their side effects are less familiar to many midwives and doctors and on the rare occasion that they appear, their significance may be overlooked.

In parturients considered to be at increased risk of requiring caesarean section, epidural analgesia should be preferred to pethidine in part because of the gastrointestinal changes mentioned above, but also because of the rapidity with which an effective epidural block can be extended in the event of an emergency caesarean section.

In pregnancy-induced hypertension, pethidine is ineffective in preventing surges in blood pressure caused by the pain of uterine contraction. Its use may also worsen acid–base balance in an already compromised fetus.[80] Furthermore, because some anaesthetists feel that pregnancy induced hypertension is a contraindication to spinal anaesthesia because it is desirable to avoid the need for a vasopressor, failing to establish epidural analgesia in labour may commit the patient to general anaesthesia if she needs urgent caesarean section. Epidural anaesthesia is therefore accepted as the method of choice for caesarean section, hence epidural analgesia must be preferable to pethidine for pain relief in labour. Finally, pethidine is unsuitable for use in severe pregnancy-induced hypertension because its active metabolite, norpethidine, has been shown in non-pregnant patients to have pro-convulsant properties.[61,81] Renal impairment, which is often associated with pregnancy-induced hypertension, reduces the clearance of norpethidine, increasing the likelihood of this complication.

Routes and modes of administration

Most commonly pethidine is administered by the intramuscular route in doses of 50–100 mg, 3–4 hourly. The site of intramuscular injection may be important as there is some evidence that absorption of pethidine from the gluteus muscle is impaired during labour and that deltoid administration may produce superior analgesia.[82] However, in an effort to try to improve the quality of analgesia, a number of other methods have been investigated.

Some studies suggest that intravenous administration is better than intramuscular. In a randomised controlled study, Isenor *et al* compared a group of women given 50–100 mg of pethidine every 2 hours as required with a group receiving an initial intravenous bolus of 25 mg followed by a continuous infusion of 60 mg/h with intermittent boluses of 25 mg/h as required. Both groups were limited to a maximum total dose of 200 mg. The intravenous group reported significantly lower pain scores with no differences in maternal or neonatal complications, although they received significantly higher doses of pethidine.[83]

The use of patient controlled analgesia (PCA) has been reported to be superior by some authors but of little benefit and potentially more dangerous to mother and newborn by others.[84,85] Robinson et al showed that women given intermittent intramuscular injections of 150 mg received more pethidine than those allowed to self-administer intermittent intravenous boluses of 0·25 mg/kg at 10 minute intervals.[84] On the other hand, Rayburn et al compared nurse administration of 25–50 mg 3-hourly with patient controlled intermittent doses of 10 mg (after 20 mg loading dose) and claimed that pain relief was equivalent in the two groups. There was an increase in the incidence of neonatal depression in the PCA group associated with the larger maternal dose.[86] Li et al looked at the feasibility of using intramuscular PCA in a small study comparing meptazinol and pethidine used via this route, but it is unlikely that this technique will confer any significant advantage.[87]

In summary, although some techniques of systemic opioid administration may confer marginal benefits, overall quality of analgesia remains poor and the wide spectrum of unpleasant side effects is largely unaltered.

Alternative opioids

Pethidine is the most widely used opioid in the UK (see Table 5.4), as in many countries. Many alternatives to pethidine have been investigated over the years. The aim has been to try to reduce the side effects and to improve the analgesia. Although several alternatives have drawn a small number of enthusiastic supporters, this enthusiasm has been based only on anecdotal reports.

Morphine and diamorphine

Morphine was probably the first opioid to be used as an analgesic in labouring women.[1] However, it fell from favour in the first half of the twentieth century, in part because of its association with "twilight sleep", and in part because its dangerous addictive side effects were well recognised. When pethidine was first introduced it was mistakenly supposed to be a safer substitute and it was thought that its higher lipid solubility might improve its efficacy. In more recent years, increasing evidence of the lack of efficacy of pethidine has led to the re-examination of the role of morphine. Olofsson et al made a careful assessment of incremental intravenous doses and demonstrated that the reduction in overall pain score measured during the first stage of labour was clinically insignificant, although there was a reduction in the number of women experiencing back pain.[21] Although they noted no neonatal side effects, they observed profound sedation in the mothers. In another recent study the same group compared pethidine and morphine.[22] Both groups of parturients continued to report high pain scores despite intravenous drug administration in well judged doses. The use of morphine conferred no advantage and caused similar side effects, of which sedation was particularly prominent (see Figure 5.3).

Though systemic diamorphine is used enthusiastically in a small number of units, there is little information comparing it with other opioids, though many studies relate its use for regional analgesia. Its increased lipid solubility suggests that it might reach the sites of action more quickly than morphine, but there is no information about its efficacy or side effect profile compared with pethidine or morphine.

Meptazinol

Meptazinol is a mixed opioid agonist/antagonist, primarily at the κ receptor, with some cholinergic effects. It enjoys popularity in a small number of units (see Table 5.4), where it is believed to be superior to pethidine (but see below). It is given in doses of 100–150 mg i.m. every 2–4 hours, having approximately one-tenth the potency of morphine and a slightly shorter duration of action. In high doses it has dysphoric side effects which reduce its potential for abuse, and its antagonist properties may cause withdrawal in parturients dependent on μ agonists. It has a reduced potential to cause respiratory depression. There is some theoretical concern that any respiratory depression it does cause may be only partially reversed by naloxone, although this has never been reported in obstetric use.

Morrison et al compared pethidine with meptazinol in a prospective randomised double blind study of 1100 parturients.[88] Both groups received the same dose of either drug, 100 mg for parturients weighing less than 70 kg and 150 mg for those weighing more. They reported no difference in analgesia or neonatal outcome but an increase in maternal vomiting with meptazinol. They noted that the most striking findings were the poor quality of pain relief in both groups and the high incidence of side effects. Other groups reported only minor if any differences in analgesia with meptazinol compared to pethidine.[89–91] It has been suggested that the half-life of meptazinol in the newborn is shorter than that of pethidine.[92] However, de Boer et al noted that although neonatal respiratory depression as evidenced by acid–base data was less at 10 minutes after delivery, this was no longer apparent at 60 minutes.[93]

Pentazocine

Pentazocine is a mixed μ agonist/antagonist and a κ and σ agonist of about one-third the potency of morphine, that enjoyed popularity in the early 1970s. As with many such opioids, it was deliberately synthesised to minimise its potential for abuse – large doses causing dysphoric side effects. It is presented as a racemic mixture of which the l-isomer alone has analgesic activity mediated through the $κ_1$ receptor. Although it does cause some sedation, there is a ceiling to this effect at larger doses. It is irritant on intramuscular or subcutaneous administration. For analgesia in labour it was given in a dose of 40 mg i.m. every 2–4 hours.

In 1966 Filler *et al* demonstrated that pentazocine had no effect on fetal heart rate, did not delay the progress of labour and may actually have accelerated labour in some cases.[43] Pentazocine grew in popularity over the next few years because, although it did not provide superior analgesia to pethidine, it appeared to cause fewer side effects in mother and baby – most notably maternal emesis.[94–98] It fell from favour quite rapidly, however, because it was relatively short-acting and repeated doses provided diminishing analgesia and occasional dysphoria.

Nalbuphine

Nalbuphine is a mixed μ agonist/antagonist and a κ agonist with clinical effects similar to pentazocine. It is a more potent μ antagonist than pentazocine but causes analgesia mediated primarily by the κ receptor. It is approximately equipotent to morphine and is given in doses of 10–20 mg i.m. in labour. Once again, its perceived advantage is that as a competitive antagonist it has a ceiling effect and might therefore be less likely to cause excessive maternal or fetal respiratory depression. However κ-mediated sedation is a common side effect and it can cause dysphoria, though less so than pentazocine.[99]

Dan *et al* compared the intravenous administration of 10 mg nalbuphine with 50 mg pethidine and showed little difference in analgesia or side effects, although there was a suggestion of transient neonatal central nervous system depression in the nalbuphine group.[100] Wilson *et al* compared the intramuscular administration of 20 mg nalbuphine with 100 mg pethidine and demonstrated a significant reduction in neonatal neurobehavioural scores at 2–4 hours of life in the nalbuphine group but without any difference in maternal analgesia.[101] More recently, intravenous nalbuphine 10 mg was shown to produce a greater reduction in fetal heart rate variability than did pethidine 50 mg.[102] When given by i.v. PCA, nalbuphine in doses of 3 mg produced better analgesia than pethidine 15 mg but with no difference in other maternal or neonatal effects.[103] Although the administration of nalbuphine by a PCA may improve satisfaction and reduce drowsiness,[85] with no consistent improvement in analgesic efficacy and the possibility of less good neonatal outcome, nalbuphine has not found widespread poularity.

Fentanyl

Fentanyl is a highly lipid-soluble phenylpiperidine derivative acting primarily on μ receptors that is approximately 80–100 times as potent as morphine. Its lipid solubility results in a rapid onset of action, but although its duration of action is shorter due to rapid redistribution, its terminal half-life – approximately 8 hours – is longer than that of morphine or pethidine.[104] Fentanyl is principally bound to albumin, favouring transplacental transfer, and when used repeatedly during labour, fetal/maternal ratios have been shown to rise to about 0·7 or more.[104,105]

Although more commonly used and thoroughly investigated when given by the epidural or spinal routes, fentanyl has been used systemically in labour. In an unblinded study of 105 women, Rayburn et al showed that fentanyl given intravenously (50–100 μg/h) produced similar analgesia to intravenous pethidine (25–50 mg/h). Maternal nausea, vomiting and sedation were worse in the pethidine group and although neonatal side effects were reported as similar, naloxone was given more frequently in the pethidine group.[106] In a previous study, the same group had reported that intravenous fentanyl given in a cumulative dose of 50–600 μg titrated according to maternal needs to 137 women caused no hazards to mother or baby.[107] However, they did observe a transient decrease in fetal heart rate variability in the 30 minutes immediately following fentanyl administration. Unfortunately most other information about the use of systemic fentanyl in labour consists of case reports of its use in women in whom, for various reasons, epidural analgesia was contraindicated.[108,109] Although there are no prospective double blind trials comparing intravenous fentanyl with pethidine, it is unlikely that the former will provide significantly better analgesia by this route.

Tramadol

Tramadol is a weak μ agonist that has been prescribed in labour in doses of 50–100 mg 4-hourly. Once again its proposed advantage was that it had been reported to have few of the detrimental side effects associated with other opioids.[110] In a randomised, double blind trial, Viegas et al reported that tramadol 100 mg was as effective as pethidine 75 mg, but that tramadol was associated with fewer maternal side effects and less respiratory depression in the newborn.[111] Conversely, Prasertsawat et al, comparing tramadol 100 mg with morphine 10 mg and pethidine 100 mg, reported no differences in either analgesia or side effects except for the fact that maternal nausea was more common with tramadol.[112]

Summary

Pethidine has been shown to provide inadequate analgesia while causing a plethora of unpleasant and potentially dangerous side effects. Its continued popularity probably results in part from its ease of administration. Despite its widespread use, serious side effects are apparently rare, though its more insidious sequelae are difficult to audit. The majority of alternative opioids provide equally inadequate analgesia while their side effect profiles differ very little. It may be that some of the shorter-acting opioids such as fentanyl or alfentanil offer slight advantages and may be appropriate in situations where regional techniques are unavailable or contraindicated, but most reports are anecdotal and more investigation is needed.

References

1 Chamberlain G. The history of pain relief in labour. In: Chamberlain G, Wraight A, Steer P, eds. *Pain and its relief in childbirth: the results of a national survey conducted by the National Birthday Trust*. Edinburgh: Churchill Livingstone, 1993:1–9.

2 Burton J. *Essay towards a complete new system of midwifery, theoretical and practical, together with several new improvements whereby women may be delivered in the most dangerous cases with more easy and safe position than has by any other method heretofore practised*. York, 1751.

3 Pitcock CD, Clark RB. From Fanny to Ferdinand: the development of consumerism in pain control during the birth process. *Am J Obstet Gynecol* 1992;3:1–8.

4 Eisleb O, Schaumann NO. Dolantin, ein neuratiges Spasmolytikum und Analgetikum (Chemisches und Pharmakologisches). *Dtsch Med Wochenschr* 1939;65:967–8.

5 Misuse of drugs regulations 1985. SI 2066, London, HMSO.

6 Martin WR, Eades CG, Thompson JA, Huppler RE, Gilbert PE. The effects of morphine- and nalorphine-like drugs in the nondependent and morphine dependent chronic spinal dog. *J Pharmacol Exp Ther* 1976;197:517–32.

7 Lord JAH, Waterfield AA, Hughes J, Kosterlitz HW. Endogenous opioid peptides: multiple agonists and receptors. *Nature* 1977;267:495–9.

8 Brownstein MJ. A brief history of opiates, opioid peptides, and opioid receptors. *Proc Natl Acad Sci USA* 1993;90:5391–3.

9 North RA, Williams JT, Surprenant A, Christie MJ. Mu and delta receptors belong to a family of receptors that are coupled to potassium channels. *Proc Natl Acad Sci USA* 1987;84:5487–91.

10 Tsunoo A, Yoshii M, Narahashi T. Block of calcium channels by enkephalin and somatostatin in neuroblastoma-glioma hybrid NG 108–15. *Proc Natl Acad Sci USA* 1986;83:9832–6.

11 Reisine T, Pasternak G. Opioid analgesia and antagonists. In: Limbird LE, Hardman JG, Molinoff PB, Rudden RW, Goodman Gilman A, eds. *The Pharmacological Basis of Therapeutics* (9th edn). New York: McGraw-Hill, 1996.

12 Reynolds F. Pharmacology of opioids. In: Van Zundert A, Ostheimer GW, eds. *Pain relief and anesthesia in obstetrics*. New York: Churchill Livingstone, 1996.

13 Oldendorf WH, Hyman S, Braun L, Oldendorf SZ. Blood–brain barrier: penetration of morphine, codeine, heroin and methadone after carotid injection. *Science* 1972;**178**: 984–6.

14 Krauer B, Dayer P, Anner R. Changes in serum albumin and alpha-1 acid glycoprotein concentrations during pregnancy: an analysis of feto-maternal pairs. *Br J Obstet Gynaecol* 1984;**91**:875–81.

15 Kuhnert BR, Kuhnert PM, Philipson EH *et al.* Disposition of meperidine and normeperidine following multiple doses during labor. II. Fetus and neonate. *Am J Obstet Gynecol* 1985;**151**:410–15.

16 Basbaum AL, Fields HL. Endogenous pain control systems: brainstem spinal pathways. *Ann Rev Neurosci* 1984;**7**:309–38.

17 Justins DM, Knott C, Luthman J, Reynolds F. Epidural versus intramuscular fentanyl. Analgesia and pharmacokinetics in labour. *Anaesthesia* 1983;**38**:937–42.

18 Oldroyd GJ, Tham EJ, Power I. An investigation into the local anaesthetic effects of pethidine in volunteers. *Anaesthesia* 1994;**49**:503–6.

19 Steer P. The methods of pain relief used. In: Chamberlain G, Wraight A, Steer P, eds. *Pain and its relief in childbirth: the results of a national survey conducted by the National Birthday Trust.* London: Churchill Livingstone, 1993:49–67.

20 Barnes J. Pethidine in labour: results in 500 cases. *BMJ* 1947;**5**:437–52.

21 Olofsson C, Ekblom A, Ekman-Ordeberg G, Granstrom L, Irestedt L. Analgesic efficacy of intravenous morphine in labour pain: a reappraisal. *Int J Obstet Anesth* 1996;**5**:176–80.

22 Olofsson C, Ekblom A, Ekman-Ordeberg G, Hjelm A, Irestedt L. Lack of analgesic effect of systemically administered morphine or pethidine on labour pain. *Br J Obstet Gynaecol* 1996;**103**:968–72.

23 Morgan BM, Bulpitt CJ, Clifton P, Lewis PJ. The consumers' attitude to obstetric care. *Br J Obstet Gynaecol* 1984;**91**:624–8.

24 Holdcroft A, Morgan M. An assessment of the analgesic effect in labour of pethidine and 50% nitrous oxide in oxygen (Entonox). *J Obstet Gynaecol Br Commonw* 1974;**81**: 603–7.

25 Harrison RF, Shore M, Woods T, Mathews G, Gardiner J, Unwin A. A comparative study of transcutaneous electrical nerve stimulation (TENS), Entonox, pethidine + promazine and lumbar epidural for pain relief in labor. *Acta Obstet Gynecol Scand* 1987;**66**:9–14.

26 Ranta P, Jouppila P, Spalding M, Kangas-Saarela T, Hollmen A, Jouppila R. Parturients' assessment of water blocks, pethidine, nitrous oxide, paracervical and epidural blocks in labour. *Int J Obstet Anesth* 1994;**3**:193–8.

27 Thorp JA, Hu DH, Albin RM, McNitt J, Meyer BA, Cohen GR *et al.* The effect of intrapartum epidural analgesia on nulliparous labor: a randomized controlled, prospective trial. *Am J Obstet Gynecol* 1993;**169**:851–8.

28 Walker JJ, Johnston J, Fairlie FM, Lloyd J, Bullingham R. A comparative study of intramuscular ketorolac and pethidine in labour pain. *Eur J Obstet Gynecol Reprod Biol* 1992;**46**:87–94.

29 Ramin SM, Gambling DR, Lucas MJ, Sharma SK, Sidawi JE, Leveno KJ. Randomized trial of epidural versus intravenous analgesia during labor. *Obstet Gynecol* 1995;**86**:783–9.

30 Robinson JO, Rosen M, Evans JM, Revill SI, David H, Rees GAD. Maternal opinion about analgesia for labour. A controlled trial between epidural block and intramuscular pethidine combined with inhalation. *Anaesthesia* 1980;**35**:1173–81.

31 Schwickerath J, Wolff F. Opiate analgesia in labour – use of nalbuphine in comparison with administration of the combination Dolantin/Atosil/Haldol. *Geburtschilfe Frauenheilkunde* 1991;**51**:897–900.

32 Rosenblatt WH, Cioffi AM, Sinatra R, Saberski LR, Silverman DG. Metoclopramide: an analgesic adjunct to patient controlled analgesia. *Anesth Analg* 1991;**73**:553–5.

33 Lisander B. Evaluation of the analgesic effect of metoclopramide after opioid-free analgesia. *Br J Anaesth* 1993;**70**:631–3.

34 Vella L, Francis D, Houlton P, Reynolds F. (1985) Comparison of the antiemetics metoclopramide and promethazine in labour. *BMJ* 1985;**290**:1173–5.

35 Nimmo WS, Wilson J, Prescott LF. Narcotic analgesia and delayed gastric emptying during labour. *Lancet* 1975;**i**:890–3.

36 Holdsworth JD. Relationship between stomach contents and analgesia in labour. *Br J Anaesth* 1978;**50**:1145–8.

37 Murphy DF, Nally B, Gardiner J, Unwin A. Effect of metoclopramide on gastric emptying before elective and emergency caesarean section. *Br J Anaesth* 1984;**56**:113–16.

38 Vanner RG. Gastro-oesophageal reflux and regurgitation during general anaesthesia for termination of pregnancy. *Int J Obstet Anesth* 1992;**1**:123–8.

39 Department of Health. *Changing Childbirth*. London: HMSO, 1993.

40 Huch R. Maternal hyperventilation and the fetus. *J Perin Med* 1986;**14**:3–17.

41 Reed PN, Colquhoun AD, Hanning CD. Maternal oxygenation during normal labour. *Br J Anaesth* 1989;**62**:316–18.

42 Griffin RP, Reynolds F. Maternal hypoxaemia during labour and delivery: the influence of analgesia and the effect on neonatal outcome. *Anaesthesia* 1995;**50**:151–6.

43 Filler WW, Filler MW. Effect of a potent non-narcotic analgesic agent (pentazocine) on uterine contraction and fetal heart rate. *Obstet Gynecol* 1966;**28**:224–32.

44 Russell JA, Gosden RG, Humphreys EM, *et al.* Interruption of parturition in rats by morphine: a result of inhibition of oxytocin secretion. *J Endocrinol* 1989;**121**:521–36.

45 Russell JA, Leng G, Coombes JE, Crockett SA, Douglas AJ, Murray I, Way S. Pethidine (meperidine) inhibition of oxytocin secretion and action in parturient rats. *Am J Physiol* 1991;**261**:R358–R368.

46 Lindow SW, van der Spuy ZM, Hendricks MS, Rosselli AP, Lombard C, Leng G. The effect of morphine and naloxone administration on plasma oxytocin concentrations in the first stage of labour. *Clin Endocrinol* 1992;**37**:349–53.

47 Bicknell RJ, Leng G, Russell JA, Dyer RG, Mansfield S, Zhao BG. Hypothalamic opioid mechanisms controlling oxytocic neurones during parturition. *Brain Res Bull* 1988;**20**:743–9.

48 Thornton S, Charlton L, Murray BJ, Davison JM, Bayliss PH. The effect of early labour, maternal analgesia and fetal acidosis on fetal plasma oxytocin levels. *Br J Obstet Gynaecol* 1993;**100**:425–9.

49 Landon MJ, Copes DR, Shiells EA, Davison GM. Degradation of radiolabelled vasopressin (125I-AVP) by the human placenta perfused in vitro. *Br J Obstet Gynaecol* 1988;**95**:488–92.

50 Pajntar M, Vlentincic B, Verdenik I. The effect of pethidine hydrochloride on the cervical muscles in the active phase of labour. *Clin Exp Obstet Gynecol* 1993;**X**:145–50.

51 Milwidsky A, Finci-Yeheskel Z, Mayer M. Direct stimulation of urokinase, plasmin and collagenase by meperidine: a possible mechanism for the ability of meperidine to enhance cervical effacement and dilation. *Am J Perinatol* 1993;**10**:130–4.

52 Reynolds F. Placental transfer of opioids. In: Budd K, ed. Update in opioids. *Clini Anaesthesiol* 1987;**1**:859–81.

53 Hamshaw-Thomas A, Reynolds F. Placental transfer of bupivacaine, pethidine and lignocaine in the rabbit. Effect of umbilical flow rate and protein content. *Br J Obstet Gynaecol* 1985;**92**:706–13.

54 Gaylard DG, Carson RJ, Reynolds F. The effect of umbilical perfusate pH and controlled maternal hypotension on placental drug transfer in the rabbit. *Anesth Analg* 1990;**71**:42–8.

55 Shnider S, Moya F. Effects of meperidine on the newborn infant. *Am J Obstet Gynecol* 1964;**89**:1009–15.

56 Belfrage P, Boreus LO, Hartvig P *et al.* Neonatal depression after obsterical analgesia with pethidine: the role of the injection–delivery time interval and of the plasma concentrations of pethidine and norpethidine. *Acta Obstet Gynecol Scand* 1981;**60**:43–9.

57 Crawford JS and Rudofsky S. Some alterations in the pattern of drug metabolism associated with pregnancy, oral contraception and the newly-born. *Br J Anaesth* 1966;**38**:446–54.

58 Kuhnert BR, Kuhnert PM, Tu ASL *et al.* Meperidine and normeperidine levels following meperidine administration in labor. I. Mother. *Am J Obstet Gynecol* 1979;**133**:904–8.

59 O'Donoghue SEF. Distribution of pethidine and chlorpromazine in maternal, fetal and neonatal biological fluids. *Nature* 1971;**229**:124–5.

60 Golub MS, Eisele JH, Kuhnert BR. Disposition of intrapartum narcotic analgesics in monkeys. *Anesth Analg* 1988;**67**:637–43.

61 Pryle BJ, Grech H, Stoddart PA, O'Mahoney T, Carson RJ, Reynolds F. (1992) The toxicity of norpethidine in sickle cell crisis. *BMJ* 1992;**304**:1478–9.

62 Kariniemi V, Ammala P. Effects of intramuscular pethidine on fetal heart variability during labour. *Br J Obstet Gynaecol* 1981;**88**:718–20.

63 Yeh SY, Forsythe A, Hon EH. Quantification of fetal heart beat to beat interval differences. *Obstet Gynecol* 1973;**41**:355–63.

64 Zimmer EZ, Divon MY, Vadasz A. Influence of meperidine on fetal movements and heart rate beat-to-beat variability in the active phase of labor. *Am J Perinatol* 1981;**5**: 197–200.

65 Rosen MG, Scibetta JJ, Hochberg CJ. Human fetal EEG III: pattern changes in the presence of fetal heart rate alterations and after use of maternal medication. *Obstet Gynecol* 1970;**361**:132–40.

66 Baxi LV, Petrie RH, James LS. Human fetal oxygenation (tcPo₂), heart rate variability and uterine activity following maternal administration of meperidine. *J Perin Med* 1988; **16**:23–30.

67 Thalme B, Belfrage P, Raabe N. Lumbar epidural analgesia in labour I: acid-base balance and clinical condition of the mother, fetus and newborn child. *Acta Obstet Gynecol Scand* 1974;**53**:27–35.

68 Taylor ES, von Fumetti HH, Essig EL, Goodman SN, Walker LC. The effects of demerol and trichloroethylene on arterial oxygen saturation in the newborn. *Am J Obstet Gynecol* 1955;**69**:348–51.

69 Koch G, Wendel H. Effect of pethidine on the post natal adjustment of respiration and acid-base balance. *Acta Obstet Gynecol Scand* 1968;**47**:27–37.

70 Hamza J, Benlabed M, Orhant E, Escourrou P, Curzi-Dascalova L, Gaultier C. Neonatal pattern of breathing during active and quiet sleep after maternal administration of meperidine. *Pediatr Res* 1992;**32**:412–16.

71 Emde RN, Swedberg J, Suzudi B. Human wakefulness and biological rhythms after birth. *Arch Gen Psychiatry* 1975;**32**:780–3.

72 Nissen E, Lilja G, Matthiesen AS Ransjo-Arvidson AB, Uvnas-Moberg K, Widstrom AM. Effects of maternal pethidine on infants' developing breast feeding behaviour. *Acta Paediatr* 1995;**84**:140–5.

73 Weiner PC, Hogg MI, Rosen M. Neonatal respiration, feeding and neurobehavioural state. *Anaesthesia* 1979;**34**:996–1004.

74 Bernard ED, Cross KW. Rectal temperature in the newborn after birth asphyxia. *BMJ* 1958;**2**:1197–9.

75 Moreland TA, Brice JEH, Walker CHM, Parija AC. Naloxone pharmacokinetics in the newborn. *Br J Clin Pharmacol* 1980;**9**:609–12.

76 Weiner PC, Hogg MJ, Rosen M. Effects of naloxone on pethidine induced neonatal depression. *BMJ* 1977;**2**:228–31.

77 Weiner PC, Wallace S. Effects of naloxone on pethidine induced neonatal depression (Letter). *BMJ* 1980;**280**:252.

78 Jacobsen B, Nyberg K, Gronbladh L *et al.* Opiate addiction in adult offspring through possible imprinting after obstetric treatment. *BMJ* 1990;**301**:1067–70.

79 Jaffee JB, Drease GE, Kelly T, Newman LM. Severe respiratory depression in the obstetric patient after intrathecal meperidine or sufentanil. *Int J Obstet Anesth* 1997;**6**: 182–4.

80 Kariniemi V, Rosti J. Intramuscular pethidine during labour associated with metabolic acidosis in the newborn. *J Perinat Med* 1986;**14**:131–5.

81 Stone PA, Macintyre PE, Jarvis DA. Norpethidine toxicity and patient controlled analgesia. *Br J Anaesth* 1993;**71**:738–40.

82 Lazebnik N, Kuhnert BR, Carr PC, Brashear WT, Syracuse CD, Mann LI. Intravenous, deltoid, or gluteus administration of meperidine during labor? *Am J Obstet Gynecol* 1989; **160**:1184–9.

83 Isenor L, Penny-MacGillivray T. Intravenous meperidine infusion for obstetric analgesia. *J Obstet Gynecol Neonatal Nurs* 1993;**22**:349–56.
84 Robinson JO, Rosen M, Evans JM, Revill SI, David H, Rees G. Self-administered intravenous and intramuscular pethidine. A controlled trial in labour. *Anaesthesia* 1980; **35**:763–70.
85 Podlas J, Breland BD. Patient controlled analgesia with nalbuphine during labor. *Obstet Gynecol* 1987;**70**:202–4.
86 Rayburn W, Leuschen MP, Earl R, Woods M, Lokovic M, Gaston-Johansson F. Intravenous meperidine during labor: a randomized comparison between nurse and patient controlled administration. *Obstet Gynecol* 1989;**74**:702–6.
87 Li DF, Rees GA, Rosen M. Feasibility of self-administration analgesia by the intramuscular route in labour. *Eur J Obstet Gynecol Reprod Biol* 1988;**27**:99–104.
88 Morrison CE, Dutton D, Howie H, Gilmour H. Pethidine compared with meptazinol during labour. A prospective randomised double-blind study in 1100 patients. *Anaesthesia* 1987;**42**:7–14.
89 Osler M. A double blind comparison of meptazinol and pethidine for pain relief in labour. *Eur J Obstet Gynecol Reprod Biol* 1987;**26**:15–18.
90 Sheikh A, Tunstall ME. Comparative study of meptazinol and pethidine for the relief of pain in labour. *Br J Obstet Gynaecol* 1986;**93**:264–9.
91 Nichol ADG, Robson PJ. Double blind comparison of meptazinol and pethidine in labour. *Br J Obstet Gynaecol* 1982;**89**:318–22.
92 Jackson MBA, Robson PJ. Preliminary clinical and pharmokinetic experiences in the new born when meptazinol is compared with pethidine as an obstetric analgesic. *Postgrad Med J* 1983;**59**:47–51.
93 de Boer FC, Shortland D, Simpson RL, Clifford WA, Catley DM. A comparison of the effects of maternally administered meptazinol and pethidine on neonatal acid–base status. *Br J Obstet Gynaecol* 1987;**94**:256–61.
94 Mowat J, Garrey MM. Comparison of pentazocine and pethidine in labour. *BMJ* 1970; **2**:757–9.
95 Moore J, Carson RM, Hunter RJ. A comparison of the effects of pentazocine and pethidine administered during labour. *J Obstet Gynaecol Br Commonw* 1970;**77**:830–6.
96 Moolgaoker AS, Cruse PM. The relief of pain in labour. A comparison of pentazocine (Fortral) and pethidine. *Clin Trials J* 1972;**9**:3–10.
97 Moore J, Ball HG. A sequential study of intravenous analgesic treatment during labour. *Br J Anaesth* 1974;**46**:365–72.
98 Refstadt SO, Lindbaek L. Ventilatory depression of the newborn of women receiving pethidine or pentazocine. A double-blind comparative trial. *Br J Anaesth* 1980;**52**:265–71.
99 Mitterschiffthaler G, Huter O. [Pethidine or nalbuphine for obstetric analgesia?] [German] *Geburtshilfe Frauenheilkunde* 1991;**51**:362–5.
100 Dan U, Rabinovici Y, Barkai G, Modan M, Etchin A, Mashiach S. Intravenous pethidine and nalbuphine during labor: a prospective double blind study. *Gynecol Obstet Invest* 1991;**32**:39–43.
101 Wilson CM, McClean E, Moore J, Dundee JW. A double blind comparison of intramuscular pethidine and nalbuphine in labour. *Anaesthesia* 1986;**41**:1207–13.
102 Giannina G, Guzman ER, Lai YL, Lake MF, Cernadas M, Vintzileos AM. Comparison of the effects of meperidine and nalbuphine on intrapartum fetal heart rate tracings. *Obstet Gynecol* 1995;**86**:441–5.
103 Frank M, McAteer EJ, Cattermole R, Loughnan B, Stafford LB, Hitchcock AM. Nalbuphine for obstetric analgesia. A comparison of nalbuphine with pethidine for pain relief in labour when administered by patient-controlled analgesia (PCA). *Anaesthesia* 1987;**42**:697–703.
104 Shafer SL, Varvel JR. Pharmacokinetics, pharmacodynamics and rational opioid selection. *Anesthesiology* 1991;**74**:53–63.
105 Ewah B, Yau K, King M, Reynolds F, Carson RJ, Morgan B. Effects of opioids on gastric emptying in labor. *Int J Obstet Anesth* 1993;**2**:125–8.

111

106 Rayburn WF, Smith CV, Parriot JE, Woods RE. Randomized comparison of meperidine and fentanyl during labor. *Obstet Gynecol* 1989;**74**:604–6.
107 Rayburn WF, Rathke A, Leuschen MP, Chleborad J, Weidner W. Fentanyl citrate analgesia during labor. *Am J Obstet Gynecol* 1989;**161**:202–6.
108 Rosaeg OP, Kitts JB, Koren G, Byford LJ. Maternal and fetal effects of intravenous patient-controlled fentanyl analgesia during labour in a thrombocytopenic parturient. *Can J Anaesth* 1992;**39**:277–81.
109 Kleiman SJ, Wiesel S, Tessler MJ. Patient controlled analgesia (PCA) using fentanyl in a parturient with a platelet function abnormality. *Can J Anaesth* 1991;**38**:489–91
110 Huber HP. Psychologic test of activity of new analgesic of the cyclohexanol series. *Arzneim-Forsch Drug Res* 1979;**28**:189.
111 Viegas OAC, Khaw B, Ratnam SS. Tramadol in labour pain in primiparous patients. A prospective comparative clinical trial. *Eur J Obstet Gynecol Reprod Biol* 1993;**49**:131–5.
112 Prasertsawat PO, Herabutya, Y, Chaturachinda K. Obstetric analgesia: comparison between tramadol, morphine and pethidine. *Curr Ther Res* 1986;**40**:1022–8.

6: Eating in labour: implications for analgesia

Background

Physiology

Effects of analgesia

Background

The choice of maternal analgesia has important implications on the safety of allowing parturients to eat during labour – a trend that is on the increase in many "progressive" delivery suites.

Before the 1940s and 1950s, very little attention was paid to the eating habits of labouring women. Undoubtedly many women laboured for hours and even days and inevitably ate and drank during their confinement. In 1946, Mendelson published his seminal work highlighting the dangers of aspiration of stomach contents during obstetric anaesthesia which resulted in a series of recommendations avidly followed by generations of obstetric

---

Mendelson's recommendations for prevention of acid aspiration in labour

- Withhold oral feeding during labour

- Increase use of local anaesthesia

- Alkalinise and empty stomach contents before induction of general anaesthesia

- Ensure competent administration of general anaesthesia

- Ensure adequate delivery room equipment, including tilting table

- Ensure anaesthetist remains with patient until laryngeal reflexes have returned

Adapted from Bogod[2]

---

anaesthetists since (see Box).[1,2] Mendelson's beliefs have been supported by the findings and recommendations presented in the Reports on Confidential

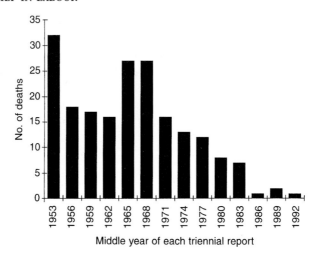

FIGURE 6.1—*Maternal mortality from pulmonary aspiration. Data taken from the triennial reports on Confidential Enquiries into Maternal Deaths in England and Wales, 1952–1984 and United Kingdom, 1985–1993*

Enquiries into Maternal Deaths covering the years from 1952 onwards. These same reports have documented a clear decline in the number of maternal deaths associated with aspiration since that time (Figure 6.1), suggesting that strict nil by mouth policies may be beneficial. More recently, these beliefs have begun to be challenged by mothers, midwives, obstetricians and even some obstetric anaesthetists.[3–6] They argue that prolonged fasting has never been scientifically proved to influence pulmonary aspiration and that since most maternal anaesthetic deaths are now caused by difficult/failed intubation in the hands of inexperienced anaesthetists, it is illogical to continue to make women fast during labour. Moreover, the metabolic consequences of fasting might even be detrimental to the progress of labour.[7–9] The Report of the Expert Maternity Group entitled "Changing Childbirth" published in 1993 placed strong emphasis on maternal choice and stipulated that within a period of 5 years providers should have been able to demonstrate a shift towards a more community-orientated service.[10] These government-backed changes will inevitably mean that many mothers will choose to consume food and drink irrespective of the dictates of the obstetric anaesthetist.

There is no doubt that a number of other changes in obstetric anaesthesia have occurred over the past 40 years, and many argue that these are of greater importance in the reduction in aspiration-related deaths than are nil by mouth policies. The development and increase in use of regional anaesthesia could have been expected to reduce the incidence of maternal aspiration. However, as Brown and Russell have shown, although the use

114

of regional anaesthesia has grown, with increasing numbers of caesarean section the absolute number of emergency caesarean sections under general anaesthesia has changed little.[11] Despite this, the absolute number of deaths from aspiration in this group has declined. Techniques of rapid sequence induction and intubation have contributed in preventing aspiration but, as the Maternal Mortality Reports demonstrate, they have introduced the complication of failed intubation. Arguments continue to rage over the influence of antacid therapy and the use of H_2 receptor antagonists, but there can be little debate over the benefit of using experienced anaesthetists in the delivery suite.

At the 1995 annual meeting of the Obstetric Anaesthetists Association, a survey of those attending suggested that over 30% of labour wards now allowed some if not all mothers to eat and drink in labour. As this fashion continues to grow it is important to address the implications this has for the provision of analgesia to labouring mothers.

Physiology

Rate of gastric emptying

It is widely accepted that from the middle of pregnancy onwards, a pregnant woman is at increased risk of aspiration should she require general anaesthesia. For a long time it was believed that delay in gastric emptying contributed to this problem.[12] More recently evidence has emerged that rate of gastric emptying is not delayed in either the second or third trimester.[13] It is now becoming clear, however, that prolonged labour does, of itself, delay gastric emptying.[14,15] Residual gastric volumes of up to 600 ml have been measured in mothers allowed a light low-fat diet during labour.[15] These volumes may constitute a risk of pulmonary aspiration should general anaesthesia be necessary during labour.

Gastro-oesophageal reflux

Both in pregnancy and during labour, physiological changes occur that increase the likelihood of gastro-oesophageal reflux. It is this effect that is undoubtedly the primary reason why pregnant women are at increased risk of aspiration. It is unclear how long this effect may last into the puerperium, although Vanner and Goodman have suggested that there is significant return to normal within 36 hours of delivery.[16]

The tendency to reflux lies in the difference between lower oesophageal sphincter pressure and intragastric pressure, the so-called "barrier pressure". Intragastric pressure rises steadily during the course of pregnancy as a result of the increasing size of the gravid uterus. At the same time,

115

lower oesophageal sphincter tone declines as a result of high circulating progesterone levels, resulting in an overall decrease in barrier pressure and a steady increase in the incidence of reflux throughout the course of pregnancy.[17]

Effects of analgesia

Supportive, non-invasive techniques and nitrous oxide

There is very little information on the effect these techniques have on the rate of gastric emptying during labour, though the findings of Holdsworth suggest they have little influence.[18] What is clear from a number of studies is that their ability to provide effective analgesia is limited.[19-22] Labouring mothers who use these techniques, along with those who choose no analgesia at all, tend to be reluctant to eat anything once they are in active labour and this to some degree lessens the problem. However, since some may have eaten in early labour, investigation is needed to explore any detrimental effects on gastric emptying that would compound the delaying effect of labour itself.

Systemic opioids

Systemic opioid administration is now recognised to be the main cause of delayed gastric emptying in labouring mothers. Nimmo *et al* demonstrated this indirectly using a paracetamol absorption technique.[23] In a study directly measuring total residual gastric volume in labouring women requiring emergency caesarean section, Holdsworth demonstrated a large increase in those who had received pethidine compared to other forms of analgesia.[18] As systemic opioids are largely ineffective at producing pain relief, however, persistent pain commonly ensures that these women are disinclined to eat in active labour. This combined with the propensity of opioids to cause vomiting may reduce the likelihood of aspiration in some individuals. However, in the majority gastric volumes are likely to be increased and furthermore any food that may have been eaten in early labour will be much more likely to remain in the stomach. This increases the danger of aspiration of solids which was the only cause of maternal *death* in Mendelson's original report.[1]

A second major consideration in women who have chosen systemic opioids for analgesia is that if they need emergency caesarean section, they are more likely to require general anaesthesia. Though in many cases general anaesthesia can be avoided by using spinal anaesthesia, this group often contains women reluctant to have regional anaesthesia of any type.

116

In summary, the use of systemic opioid analgesia is a contraindication to allowing eating during labour. Furthermore, if a woman has decided that a systemic opioid is her analgesic technique of choice, she should be strongly discouraged from eating in early labour, even before she has received any opioid. Whenever a parturient is given systemic pethidine it should, of course, be accompanied by metoclopramide, both to diminish emesis and to promote gastric emptying, and an H_2 antagonist to diminish gastric secretion, but these cannot guarantee to remove the danger.

Regional analgesia

Regional analgesia during labour using local anaesthetic alone has been shown to have no effect on gastric emptying, as assessed by paracetamol absorption, over and above the delaying effect of labour itself.[24] However, the introduction of epidural and spinal opioids in combination with bupivacaine may have reintroduced opioid-mediated delays in gastric emptying. Ewah et al demonstrated that bolus epidural doses of as little as 50 µg of fentanyl delay gastric emptying.[25] More recently, Porter et al reported that epidural fentanyl given by infusion rather than by bolus, did not prolong gastric emptying.[14]

Undoubtedly the most important implication of the use of regional analgesia in labour is that, because it provides effective analgesia, many women choosing this technique, if allowed, may continue to eat significant amounts of food throughout labour, including the second stage. This has been shown to result in significantly greater residual gastric volumes than in women allowed water only during labour.[15] On the other hand, those allowed to eat had lower levels of ketones which some have suggested may be of benefit to the progress and outcome of labour. Moreover, women with effective regional analgesia are less likely to require general anaesthesia for operative intervention. One argument put forward by those who would allow women to eat in labour is that it is natural for them to do so.[26] It is somewhat ironic that regional analgesia provides pain relief of such quality that it appears to prevent the natural tendency for women to fast once in established labour. It is for this reason that extreme caution should be exercised and more investigation is required to produce safe eating policies for labouring women who choose this form of analgesia.

References

1 Mendelson CL. The aspiration of stomach contents into the lungs during obstetric anesthesia. *Am J Obstet Gynecol* 1946;**52**:191–205.
2 Bogod DG. Gastric emptying and feeding in labour. *Curr Anaesth Crit Care* 1995;**6**:224–8.
3 Ludka LM, Roberts CC. Eating and drinking in labour. *J Nurse–Midwifery* 1993;**38**: 199–207.
4 Pengelley L, Gyte G. Eating and drinking in labour. *New Generation Digest* 1996;**13**:4–13.

117

5 Elkington KW. At the water's edge: where obstetrics and anesthesia meet. *Obstet Gynecol* 1991;**77**:304–8.
6 Bogod DG, Smith ID. Feeding in labour. *Ballières Clin Anaesthesiol* 1995;**9**:735–47.
7 Ludka L. Fasting during labour. *Proceedings of International Confederation of Midwives, 21st Congress in The Hague,* 1987.
8 Metzger BE, Vileisis RA, Ramikar V, Freinkel N. "Accelerated starvation" and the skipped breakfast in late normal pregnancy. *Lancet* 1982;**i**:588–92.
9 Dumoulin JG, Foulkes JEB. Ketonuria during labour. *Br J Obstet Gynaecol* 1984;**91**:97–8.
10 Department of Health. *Changing Childbirth.* London: HMSO, 1993.
11 Brown GW, Russell IF. A survey of anaesthesia for caesarean section. *Int J Obstet Anesth* 1995;**4**:214–18
12 Davison JS, Davison MC, Hay DM. Gastric emptying time in late pregnancy and labour. *J Obstet Gynaecol Br Commonw* 1970;**77**:37–41.
13 Whitehead EM, Smith M, Dean Y, O'Sullivan G. Gastric emptying time in late pregnancy and the puerperium. *Anaesthesia* 1993;**48**:53–7.
14 Porter J, Bonello E, Reynolds F. The influence of epidural fentanyl on gastric emptying in labour (Abstract). *Int J Obstet Anesth* 1995;**4**:261.
15 Scrutton M, Lowy C, O'Sullivan G. Eating in labour: an assessment of the risks and benefits (Abstract). *Int J Obstet Anesth* 1996;**5**:145.
16 Vanner RG, Goodman NW. Gastro-oesophageal reflux in pregnancy at term and after delivery. *Anaesthesia* 1989;**44**:808–11.
17 Van Thiel DH, Gavaler JS, Shobha AB, Joshi N, Sara RK, Stremple J. Heartburn of pregnancy. *Gastroenterology* 1977;**72**:666–8.
18 Holdsworth JD. Relationship between stomach contents and analgesia in labour. *Br J Anaesth* 1978;**50**:1145–8.
19 Ranta P, Jouppila P, Spalding M, Kangas-Saarela T, Hollmen A, Jouppila R. Parturients' assessment of water blocks, pethidine, nitrous oxide, paracervical and epidural blocks in labour. *Int J Obstet Anesth* 1994;**3**:193–8.
20 Harrison R, Woods T, Shore M, Mathews G, Unwin A. Pain relief in labour using transcutaneous electrical stimulation (TENS). A TENS/TENS placebo controlled study in two parity groups. *Br J Obstet Gynaecol* 1985;**93**:739–46.
21 Holdcroft A, Morgan M. An assessment of the analgesic effect in labour of pethidine and 50% nitrous oxide in oxygen (Entonox). *J Obstet Gynaecol Br Commonw* 1974;**81**:603–7.
22 Harrison RF, Shore M, Woods T, Mathews G, Gardiner J, Unwin A. A comparative study of transcutaneous electrical nerve stimulation (TENS), entonox, pethidine + promazine and lumbar epidural for pain relief in labor. *Acta Obstet Gynecol Scand* 1987;**66**:9–14.
23 Nimmo WS, Wilson J, Prescott LF. Narcotic analgesics and delayed gastric emptying during labour. *Lancet* 1975;**i**:890–3.
24 Petring OU, Adelhof B, Erinmadsen J, Angelo H, Jelert H. Epidural anaesthesia does not delay early postoperative gastric emptying in man. *Acta Anaesth Scand* 1984;**28**:393–5.
25 Ewah B, Yau K, King M *et al.* Effect of epidural opioids on gastric emptying in labour. *Int J Obstet Anesth* 1992;**2**:125–8.
26 Lewis P. Food for thought – should women fast or feed in labour? *Mod Midwife* 1991; July/August:14–17.

Part Three
Regional analgesia

7: Neuroscientific aspects

Anatomy and physiology

Anatomy of the vertebral canal

The safe practice of regional analgesia and anaesthesia requires detailed knowledge of the anatomy of the epidural and subarachnoid spaces. This must be combined with appreciation of the nerve pathways responsible for the transmission of pain during labour.

The spinal cord and its coverings lie within the bony cavity of the vertebral canal, which begins at the foramen magnum and passes down to end at the sacral hiatus. It is bounded anteriorly by the vertebral bodies and the intervertebral discs, laterally by the pedicals and the intervertebral foramina which lie between them and posteriorly by the laminae and the ligamenta flava between them. Superior and inferior articular processes unite adjacent vertebral arches but posteriorly in the midline access can be gained to the vertebral canal via the interlaminar foramina (Figure 7.1). It is helpful to examine the lumbar spine in a skeleton and look at the shape of each interlaminar foramen in the lumbar region. In life they are filled by the ligamenta flava.

The spinous processes in the lumbar region are described as hatchet-shaped, thus the posterior surfaces, that are palpable in thin people in the midline, are much longer than the gaps between them (Figure 7.2). The gaps between the spinous processes can be increased by flexion of the spine, but if the spinous processes are hard to feel and flexion is poor it is unlikely that a needle aiming for the epidural space in the midline will hit

121

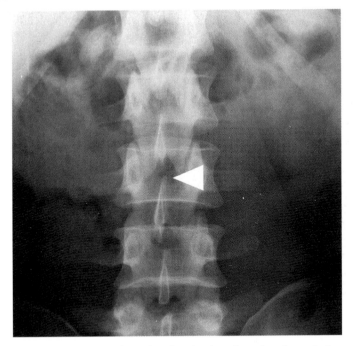

FIGURE 7.1—*AP X-ray of lumbar spine. Interlaminar foramina* (arrow) *show up dark between the spinous processes*

the gap between the spines by chance. On the other hand, a needle within the sagittal plane between the spines cannot fail to attain the interlaminar foramen.

The ligamenta flava unite in the midline to form the interspinous ligament which merges with the supraspinous ligament (Figure 7.3).

In women of childbearing age the spinal cord usually extends down to the lower border of the first lumbar vertebra. The cord and its nerve roots are covered directly with pia mater which carries the arterial supply into the nerve tissue. They are bathed in cerebrospinal fluid (CSF) which is contained within two membranes – the delicate but waterproof arachnoid mater with the tough but porous dura mater outside it. The dural sac continues down within the vertebral canal to the level of the second sacral segment. Below the termination of the cord, or conus medullaris, the sac contains the filum terminale and the closely packed lower lumbar and sacral nerve roots – the cauda equina.

The arachnoid and dural membranes lie in close approximation separated by only a film of serous fluid. The potential space between these layers can occasionally be cannulated if the dura is torn during epidural insertion.

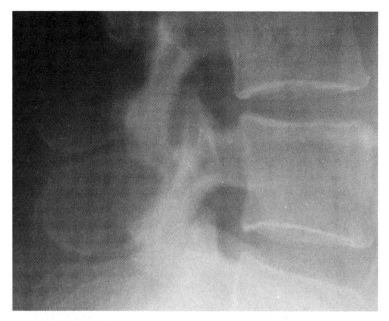

FIGURE 7.2—*Lateral X-ray of a poorly flexed lumbar spine. Note the very small gaps between the spinous processes*

The *epidural space* surrounds the dural sac within the vertebral canal. It extends from the base of the skull to the sacrococcygeal membrane and is bounded posteriorly by the ligamentum flavum on each side and anteriorly by the posterior longitudinal ligament. The space contains nerve roots, blood vessels, and fat.

The anterior part of the epidural space (the anterior epidural space) is thin containing only a small amount of fat. The two lateral spaces are segmental and each is cone-shaped and contains the nerve roots and segmental nerves. The posterior epidural space in the lumbar region is also segmental and each segment is triangular in cross-section, deepest opposite the centre of each ligamentum flavum at the midline and tapering to join the lateral space as a potential space. At the superior and inferior border each segment of the posterior space becomes only potential where the dura is in contact with the laminae.[1,2] In sagittal section (Figure 7.4), each posterior epidural space is crescentic.

The anterior and posterior spinal nerve roots cross the epidural space covered by a thin layer of meninges. The nerve roots unite at the intervertebral foramina to form the spinal nerves. The descent that each spinal nerve must make from the relevant spinal segment to the appropriate intervertebral foramen takes place almost entirely within the dural sac.

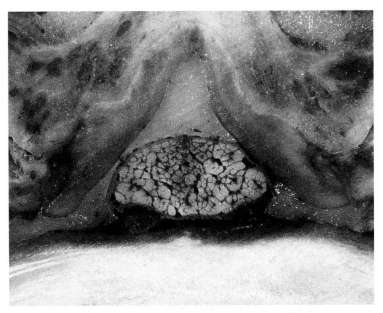

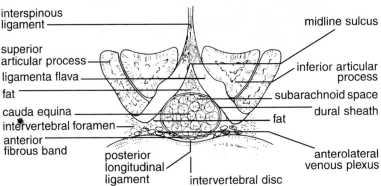

FIGURE 7.3—*Cross-section of the spinal column at the 2nd lumbar interspace. (Modified from Gaynor[3] by permission of the author and publisher)*

Fat fills the epidural space but offers little resistance to injection or the passage of an epidural catheter. Fibrous connective tissue strands connect the dural sac to the walls of the vertebral canal. It has been suggested that in certain individuals a dural fold (plica mediana dorsalis) extending to the ligamentum flavum may exist and affect the spread of epidurally administered drugs. Such a dural fold, however, has not been observed by orthopaedic surgeons at laminectomy. It may be an artefact produced by

124

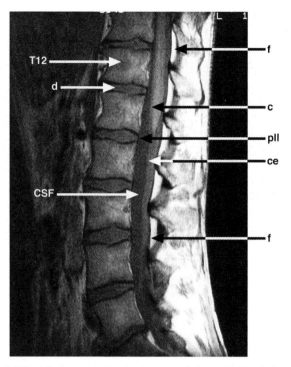

FIGURE 7.4—*MRI of the lumbar spine in the sagittal plane.* d: *disc;* f: *fat in the epidural space;* c: *conus;* pll: *posterior longitudinal ligament;* ce: *cauda equina; CSF shows up dark. (From Westbrook* et al[1] *by permission of the author and publisher)*

injection of fluid into the epidural space pushing aside the cone of fat with its midline posterior attachments. No evidence of a true plica mediana dorsalis has been found in MRI studies.[1]

Blood supply

The blood supply to the spinal cord is provided by one anterior and two posterior spinal arteries. The posterior vessels arise from the posterior inferior cerebellar arteries and the anterior is formed by branches from both vertebral arteries. The three relatively slender vessels run the entire course of the cord, receiving additional blood supply from the radicular vessels. Radicular arteries enter the epidural space through the intervertebral foramina, dividing into smaller anterior and posterior branches. The posterior branches anastomose with posterior spinal arteries providing the blood supply to the posterior part and the periphery of the cord. The main blood supply to the grey matter and the anterior part of the lower cord is from the anterior spinal artery. This is reinforced by only a few segmental

125

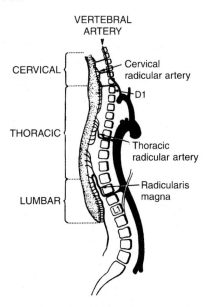

FIGURE 7.5—*The blood supply to the spinal cord, showing the three or so arteries that supplement the anterior spinal artery. (From Usubiaga[4] by permission of the publisher)*

arteries, as most anterior branches peter out before reaching the cord. The lumbar enlargement frequently relies on one radicular branch (artery of Adamkiewicz), usually arising at the lower thoracic or upper lumbar level (Figure 7.5). If this crucial artery, which is normally unilateral, is damaged, the lower part of the spinal cord may be rendered ischaemic.

Epidural veins run along the lateral walls of the spinal canal. They are connected to the systemic circulation via the internal iliac, intercostal and azygos veins and through the vertebral veins to the cerebral sinuses. The epidural veins provide an important alternative route of venous drainage from the lower half of the body during late pregnancy (see below). In the final weeks of pregnancy the epidural veins become increasingly engorged, a cause of increased spread of both epidural and spinal anaesthesia. Such venous engorgement also increases the risk of vessel puncture and inadvertent intravenous injection.

A rich supply of lymphatic vessels convey debris from the CSF out through the intervertebral foramina to reach channels in front of the vertebral bodies.

Pain pathways

Pain is conducted from the uterine body in Aδ and C fibres (see below) travelling together with sympathetic fibres grouped together to emerge on

126

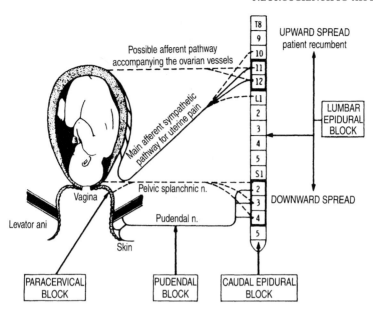

FIGURE 7.6—*Pain pathways in labour. (From Doughty[5] by permission of the author and publisher)*

either side of the uterus. They pass through the paracervical tissues and broad ligament to the sympathetic chain and enter the spinal cord via the white rami communicantes at the level of the 11th and 12th thoracic roots (Figure 7.6). There may also be a variable contribution from the 10th thoracic and 1st lumbar roots. Painful stimuli from the cervix, vagina, and perineum are transmitted by the pudendal nerve to the 2nd, 3rd, and 4th sacral roots.

Visceral pain is referred to the relevant dermatome (see Figure 3.2) and therefore uterine pain is felt across the lower abdomen and occasionally in the upper thigh. Pain felt in the upper abdomen does not have its origins in normal uterine contractions. Back pain may originate from the uterine body, the cervix or from other intrapelvic structures.

Additional nociceptive pathways are involved during caesarean section. The pain of skin incision is transmitted via the 11th and 12th thoracic roots but sensory fibres from abdominal viscera and peritoneum may enter the cord at levels up to the 5th thoracic vertebra.[6]

Nerve fibre types

An elementary understanding of the different types of fibres and how they may be affected by regional blockade is of value. Table 7.1 classifies nerve

127

TABLE 7.1—*Nerve fibre types*

Fibre type	Function	Conduction velocity (m/s)
Aα	Proprioception, somatic motor	70–120
Aβ	Touch, pressure	30–70
Aγ	Motor to muscle spindle	15–30
Aδ	Pain, temperature, touch	12–30
B	Preganglionic autonomic	3–15
C	Pain, reflex responses, postganglionic autonomic	0·5–2

fibres into the three types, depending upon their conduction speed. Large fibres conduct the most rapidly and small fibres the least. Uterine pain is carried by Aδ and to a lesser and variable extent by C fibres. The cell bodies of these sensory fibres are in the posterior root ganglion and the central projections of all C fibres and the majority of Aδ fibres synapse principally in the substantia gelatinosa, lamina II of the posterior horn. A small but variable proportion of Aδ fibres bypass this system and travel directly up in the posterior columns. Synaptic activity in the substantia gelatinosa can be inhibited presynaptically by a system of inhibitory neurones and opiate receptors which inhibit pain transmission pre- and post-synaptically, but principally by pre-synaptic inhibition of transmitter release.

Preganglionic autonomic fibres are B fibres. Sympathetic nerves that pass out of the cord in the anterior roots and pass in the white rami communicantes to the sympathetic ganglia are therefore B fibres while the postganglionic motor nerves in the autonomic nervous system are principally C fibres.

Autonomic pathways

Sympathetic fibres emerge from the spinal cord in segments T1–L2 while parasympathetics emerge via cranial nerves of which the vagus extends to the thorax and upper abdomen, and the sacral roots which supply pelvic organs. The function of the autonomic nervous system, like the somatic nervous system, is also altered by regional analgesia. The most striking effect is observed with blockade of sympathetic nerves where vasodilatation results in pooling of blood in the legs reducing venous return with a consequent fall in blood pressure.

Aorto-caval compression

The increase in the size of the pregnant uterus produces significant compression of both the inferior vena cava and the aorta when the woman lies in the supine position.[7,8] It must be stressed that by term aorto-caval compression is present in all women but in most cases venous return is maintained by flow through vertebral and paraspinous veins which drain into the azygos system. If venous return is not adequate through this collateral drainage, cardiac output is maintained by a rise in peripheral vascular resistance and to a lesser degree by an increase in heart rate. Where these compensatory mechanisms fail hypotension develops – the supine hypotensive syndrome.[8] Although fewer than 20% of women develop hypotension when supine, increased vascular resistance together with aortic compression may impair placental perfusion producing fetal acidosis. These changes may be readily overcome by turning the woman into the lateral position.

Supine hypotension is more likely to occur in the presence of regional analgesia and anaesthesia because sympathetic blockade to the lower half of the body prevents a rise in peripheral vascular resistance. It is therefore imperative that women receiving epidural or spinal blockade are never allowed to lie flat on their backs. They should be nursed in either the lateral or sitting position and if the supine position is required, for example immediately before operative delivery, adequate uterine displacement must be provided. This may be done manually or by placing a wedge under the right hip. However, these measures are not as effective in preventing supine hypotension as is the full lateral position.

Pharmacology

Increasing numbers of drugs are being investigated to find the ideal epidural or intrathecal regimen for labour analgesia. Traditionally local anaesthetics have been the most popular, but due to their potential for producing autonomic and motor block there has been a move away from high-dose to low-dose local anaesthetic solutions combined with other analgesics. Epidural and spinal opioids used alone or with low dose local anaesthetics have gained widespread acceptance. α_2-agonists such as clonidine are being investigated, as are other potential analgesics including anticholinesterases and benzodiazepines.

Local anaesthetics

Local anaesthetics prevent depolarisation and hence conduction along nerve fibres. They act on all fibre types, but Aδ and B fibres are the most sensitive, while higher doses are needed to block C fibres and the larger A fibres. Thus a low concentration of local anaesthetic placed neuraxially will readily block the element of uterine pain that is conducted by Aδ fibres and will also inhibit sympathetic nerve transmission producing anhidrosis

129

and vasodilatation. This vasodilatation will be more marked than if the local anaesthetic is placed peripheral to the sympathetic chain. Doses of local anaesthetic necessary to block all types of pain commonly lead to a degree of motor block which increases with total dose.

The overall effects that local anaesthetics have on the body may be classified as local, regional, and systemic. Local effects result from a local concentration of the drug which is one- to ten thousand-fold higher than that found systemically. Such effects are therefore not seen following systemic absorption or administration even of toxic doses. Local effects are nerve conduction block as described above and a local effect on blood vessels. While the older ester drugs procaine, amethocaine, and chloroprocaine produce vasodilatation, an amine drug such as lignocaine produces vasodilatation only at high concentration and neutral effects at low concentration.[9,10] The chiral amide local anaesthetics prilocaine, mepivacaine, and bupivacaine (those which possess an asymmetric carbon atom) are different again. The S isomer has vasoconstrictor properties and also tends to be a more potent local anaesthetic, though whether this is solely as a result of the vasoconstrictor properties is uncertain. These drugs tend to be vasoconstrictor at low concentrations as a result of the effect of the S isomer and vasodilator only at high concentrations.[11,12] Even the vasoconstrictor effect, however, depends upon a concentration higher than that which is achieved systemically even in toxic concentrations.

Regional effects result from nerve conduction blockade, and are therefore absence of sweating, vasodilatation, analgesia, numbness, loss of proprioception and motor blockade. Neuraxial administration affecting thoracic roots causes intestinal contraction and enhanced peristalsis as a result of unopposed parasympathetic activity from the vagus. Micturition is, however, dependent upon sacral parasympathetic outflow as well as sympathetic, hence blockade of sacral roots tends to cause urinary retention.

Systemic effects result from absorption of local anaesthetic from the site of administration or from accidental intravenous injection. If the onset is slow, light-headedness, dizziness, and circumoral tingling are detected initially followed by drowsiness, tremor, and, if a sufficiently large dose has been administered, generalised convulsions. Ultimately medullary depression with respiratory and circulatory arrest occurs. Doses in excess of those required to produce generalised convulsions can cause direct myocardial depression and in the case of bupivacaine convulsant doses may also cause cardiac arrhythmias.

Individual local anaesthetics

Before the advent of bupivacaine the shorter acting **lignocaine** and **mepivacaine** were used to provide epidural analgesia in labour, although the latter was not used for labour in the UK. Both had many disadvantages. They were short-acting. With lignocaine, for example, the first dose (commonly 1·5% with adrenaline) might provide analgesia for one and a half hours but tachyphylaxis was prominent and after a few doses the duration of action was often only 45 minutes.[13] Lignocaine is short-acting because, having relatively low lipid solubility, it is more rapidly absorbed than is bupivacaine from its site of administration. This absorption rate naturally exceeds elimination rate initially and plasma concentrations tend to rise to approach toxic levels before plateau concentration is reached. Hence early signs of systemic toxicity were not uncommon in mother and baby when lignocaine was used for more than just one or two doses.

With the advent of **bupivacaine** certain advantages were immediately apparent. In the early days it was commonly used by intermittent bolus in a concentration of 0·5%. A volume of 6 ml, with or without adrenaline, produced analgesia for about two hours.[14] Moreover, tachyphylaxis was not seen. The result of this reduced dose requirement was that plasma concentrations did not approach the toxic range within the duration of normal labour[15] in either mother or baby. Moreover, motor block appeared to be less prominent with bupivacaine than with lignocaine when given epidurally in analgesic doses. A disadvantage of bupivacaine is always considered to be its relative danger if given accidentally intravenously, when advantageous slow absorption no longer applies. Unlike lignocaine it can produce cardiac arrhythmias in doses near those which produce convulsions. This theoretical danger should not, however, pose a major threat provided the simple rudiments of safe practice are followed, to wit slow injection while maintaining eye contact with the patient and ensuring that early signs of inebriation are not overlooked.

Chloroprocaine is an ester local anaesthetic which is popular in the USA but is not available in the UK. It has a very rapid onset of action but an unhelpfully brief effect with an abrupt offset. It is so rapidly broken down in the plasma that it is essentially without systemic effect. It antagonises the analgesic effect of coadministered fentanyl[16] and epidural use is also associated with backache[17] which may confound the early diagnosis of epidural abscess. **Prilocaine** is not recommended as it increases methaemaglobinaemia in a dose-related manner, an effect to which the very young are highly susceptible.

Recent interest has focused on **ropivacaine**, a propyl analogue of bupivacaine and mepivacaine but presented as a single enantinomer, the S-isomer, which is more effective as a local anaesthetic than the R-isomer and has inherent vasoconstrictor properties. Epidurally it appears to be equipotent with bupivacaine in *anaesthetic* doses, a safety factor since it is less toxic. In low dose it produces less sensory and less motor block than does bupivacaine.[18]

131

Opioids (see also Chapter 5)

Opiate receptors are to be found in many areas in the brain stem and also in the spinal cord, principally in the substantia gelatinosa, lamina II of the dorsal horn. Thus opiate agonists if applied epidurally or intrathecally have ready access to these receptors at a much higher concentration than that which results from systemic administration. The effect of opiate agonism is to produce a selective block of nociceptive pathways. Opioids administered neuraxially more readily block pain transmission generated via C pain fibre stimulation than that from Aδ stimulation. It is for this reason that a successful analgesic block can be achieved in labour with low doses of a combination of opioid and local anaesthetic. Unlike local anaesthetics, however, which can act on the nerve roots within the epidural space, opioid drugs administered epidurally must first penetrate dura and arachnoid, then once in the CSF must diffuse into the substance of the cord before producing their analgesic effect.

Following epidural injection all drugs diffuse readily across the dura but penetrate the arachnoid at a rate dependent upon oil/water solubility.[19] Once in the cerebrospinal fluid, partitioning into the adjacent nervous tissue is again dependent on this property. Hence morphine which has low lipophilicity (Chapter 5) may remain for long periods in the CSF with two consequences. First, it has a slow onset and longer duration of action than other opioids. Secondly, the side effects nausea, vomiting, and respiratory depression which result from cephalad spread, may be more pronounced and longer lasting but delayed in onset. Drug clearance from the neuraxis is dependent upon blood supply, hence opioids that gain rapid access to tissues and have a rapid onset also have a shorter duration of action.

Side effects that have been reported from neuraxial opioid administration are nausea, vomiting, pruritus, urinary retention, and respiration depression. The incidence of nausea and vomiting in labour, however, is not increased by the addition of fentanyl or sufentanil to epidural bupivacaine.[20] Pruritus with agents other than morphine is unlikely to be troublesome. Urinary retention may occur anyway with plain local anaesthetics and may be minimised by the use of mobile epidurals. Equally, respiratory depression is not a major problem in the parturient who is usually young and fit and less likely to be neglected by carers than is a patient in a postoperative ward. Continuous pulse oximetry studies suggest, however, that minor degrees of maternal desaturation are more likely with epidural opioids than with plain bupivacaine infusions, particularly during the second stage of labour.[21,22] It is a sensible precaution to avoid bolus doses of neuraxial opioids in a patient who has received a systemic opioid agonist within the past 4 hours.

Individual opioid drugs (see Chapters 5 and 11)

Fentanyl has been used widely in labour in bolus doses of between 25 and 150 µg. As a sole agent it does not produce reliable analgesia throughout labour, but when combined with low dose bupivacaine it produces excellent pain relief. Epidurally, combinations varying between fentanyl 100 µg with bupivacaine 10 mg and fentanyl 30 µg with bupivacaine 15 mg all appear to provide satisfactory and reliable pain relief. The addition of fentanyl to bupivacaine provides more reliable perineal analgesia than either agent used alone.[23] Intrathecal fentanyl 25 µg with bupivacaine 2·5 mg produces rapid relief of labour pain with minimal motor block allowing mothers to ambulate during labour.[24] Epidurally, **sufentanil** in systemic equivalent doses is similar to fentanyl.[20] Larger doses of sufentanil have been used but respiratory depression is more likely.[25] Intrathecal sufentanil, in a dose of 10 µg, can be used to provide labour analgesia for over one hour.[26] **Alfentanil** has been used for epidural infusions in combination with bupivacaine. When given at a rate of 30 µg kg^{-1}min^{-1} neonatal hypotonia was observed.[27] Alfentanil 5 µg/ml added to 0·125% bupivacaine produced significantly better analgesia than did fentanyl 2 µg/ml added to bupivacaine 0·125%, with no adverse neonatal effects.[28] **Diamorphine** has a longer duration and when 5 mg was added to the epidural loading dose it reduced the requirement for bupivacaine in subsequent infusions.[29] It has also been used successfully intrathecally in doses from 0·2 mg[30] to 2·5 mg.[31] **Pethidine** owes part of its action to a local anaesthetic effect but epidural doses have a shorter duration of action than intramuscular.[32] It has been used intrathecally as sole agent for surgical procedures such as caesarean section.[33] The kappa receptor agonist **butorphanol**, when used epidurally in a dose of 3 mg, may produce somnolence in the mother[34] and a sinusoidal fetal heart trace.[35] **Morphine** when given epidurally has the capacity to produce more side effects than analgesia. As a hydrophilic opioid, it penetrates the meninges too slowly to be a useful form of labour analgesia. Nausea, vomiting, and pruritus are troublesome and compared to the lipophilic opioids, there is a much greater risk of respiratory depression. Intrathecal doses of 0·5–1 mg produce moderately good labour analgesia for 5–7 hours, but with an unacceptably slow onset of about one hour and severe side effects.[36]

Other drugs

Adrenaline and clonidine may augment analgesia produced by other agents. The α_1 action of **adrenaline** produces vasoconstriction of the epidural vessels and it intensifies the action of bupivacaine whilst prolonging that of lignocaine. Stimulation of α_2-adrenergic receptors, present in the dorsal horn, modifies the transmission of noxious sensory information by mimicking activation of descending noradrenergic pathways and inhibiting neurotransmitter release.[37] The addition of adrenaline to local anaesthetic solutions however, increases the incidence of motor block.[38] **Clonidine**, a more selective α_2-agonist than adrenaline, has been used in combination with epidural opioids and local anaesthetics to treat both labour and post-caesarean section pain.[39,40] Unlike local anaesthetics, clonidine does not enhance motor blockade or impair proprioception nor does it lead to respiratory depression, pruritus, nausea and vomiting seen with spinal opioids. It can, however, produce hypotension, bradycardia, and sedation. When combined with 0·125% bupivacaine, the optimum analgesic dose of clonidine has been reported to be 75 µg.[41] Higher doses have been studied, although there have been concerns over sedation and cardiovascular depression.[39] Epidural clonidine combined with bupivacaine does not provide better pain relief than fentanyl/bupivacaine combinations. Celleno and colleagues found little difference in the quality of analgesia between 150 µg of clonidine and 100 µg of fentanyl when added to 0·125% bupivacaine and 1:800 000 adrenaline.[42] The addition of clonidine to bupivacaine and sufentanil solutions increases the incidence of side effects whilst producing only negligible improvement in pain relief.[43]

Intrathecal injection of the anticholinesterase **neostigmine** produces analgesia in animals. Interactions between cholinergic and α_2-adrenergic systems have been investigated with spinal clonidine/neostigmine combinations.[44] By increasing activity in the sympathetic ganglia, neostigmine counteracts hypotension and bradycardia produced by spinal clonidine. However, due to its poor lipid solubility it needs to be administered well before clonidine. The more lipophilic physostigmine might prove to be a more suitable alternative.

References

1 Westbrook JL, Renowden SA, Carrie LES. Study of the anatomy of the extradural region using magnetic resonance imaging. *Br J Anaesth* 1993;**71**:495–8.

2 Capogna G, Celleno D, Simonetti C, Lupoi D. Anatomy of the lumbar epidural region using magnetic resonance imaging: a study of dimensions and comparison of two postures. *Int J Obstet Anesth* 1997;**6**:97–100.

3 Gaynor PA. The lumbar epidural region: anatomy and approach. In: Reynolds F, ed. *Epidural and spinal blockade in obstetrics*. London: Baillière Tindall, 1990:3–18.

4 Usubiaga JE. Neurological complications following epidural analgesia. *Int Anesthesiol Clin* 1975;**13**:2.

5 Doughty A. The relief of pain or labour. In: Churchill-Davidson HC, ed. *A practice of anaesthesia*, 4th edn. London: Lloyd Luke, 1978:1291.

6 Russell IF. Levels of anaesthesia and intraoperative pain at caesarean section under regional block. *Int J Obstet Anesth* 1995;**4**:71–7.

7 Marx GF. Aortocaval compression syndrome: its 50 year history. *Int J Obstet Anesth* 1992; **1**:60–4.

8 Bieniarz J, Crottogini JJ, Curuchet E *et al.* Aortocaval compression by the uterus in late human pregnancy. *Am J Obstet Gynecol* 1968;**100**:203–17.

9 Aps C, Reynolds F. The effect of concentration on vasoactivity of bupivacaine and lignocaine. *Br J Anaesth* 1976;**48**:1171–4.

10 Willatts D, Reynolds F. Comparison of the vasoactivity of amide and ester local anaesthetics: an intradermal study. *Br J Anaesth* 1985;**57**:1006.

11 Aps C, Reynolds F. An intradermal study of the local anaesthetic and vascular effects of the isomers of bupivacaine. *Br J Clin Pharmacol* 1978;**6**:63–8.

12 Fairly JW, Reynolds F. An intradermal study of the local anaesthetic and vascular effects of the isomers of mepivacaine. *Br J Anaesth* 1981;**53**:1211–16.

13 Reynolds F, Taylor G. Maternal and neonatal blood concentrations of bupivacaine. A comparison with lignocaine during continuous extradural analgesia. *Anaesthesia* 1970; **25**: 14–23.

14 Reynolds F, Taylor G. Plasma concentrations of bupivacaine during continuous epidural analgesia in labour: the effect of adrenaline. *Br J Anaesth* 1971;**43**:436–9.

15 Reynolds F, Hargrove RL, Wyman JB. Maternal and foetal plasma concentrations of bupivacaine after epidural block. *Br J Anaesth* 1973;**45**:1049–53.

16 Camann WR, Hartigan PM, Gilbertson LI, Johnson MD, Datta S. Chloroprocaine antagonism of epidural opioid analgesia: a receptor specific phenomenon? *Anesthesiology* 1990;**73**:860–3.

17 Fibuch EF, Opper SE. Back pain following epidurally administered Nesacaine-MPF. *Anesth Analg* 1989;**69**:113–15.

18 Zaric D, Nydahl P-A, Philipson L, Samuelsson L, Heierson A, Axelsson K. The effect of continuous lumbar epidural infusion of ropivacaine (0·1%, 0·2% and 0·3%) and 0·25% bupivacaine on sensory and motor block in volunteers. *Reg Anesth* 1996;**21**:14–25.

19 Bernards C, Hill HF. Morphine and alfentanil permeability through the spinal dura, arachnoid and pia mater of dogs and monkeys. *Anesthesiology* 1990;**73**:1214–19.

20 Russell R, Reynolds F. Epidural infusions for nulliparous women in labour. A randomised double blind comparison of fentanyl/bupivacaine and sufentanil/bupivacaine. *Anaesthesia* 1993;**48**:856–61.

21 Griffin RP, Reynolds F. Maternal hypoxaemia during labour and delivery: the influence of analgesia and effect on neonatal outcome. *Anaesthesia* 1995;**50**:151–5.

22 Porter JS, Benello E, Reynolds F. The effect of epidural opioids on maternal oxygenation during labour and delivery. *Anaesthesia* 1996;**51**:899–903.

23 Reynolds F, O'Sullivan G. Epidural fentanyl and perineal pain in labour. *Anaesthesia* 1989;**44**:341–4.

24 Collis RE, Davies DWL, Aveling W. Randomised comparison of combined spinal epidural and standard epidural analgesia in labour. *Lancet* 1995;**345**:1413–16.

25 Hays RL, Palmer CM. Respiratory depression after intrathecal sufentanil during labor. *Anesthesiology* 1994;**81**:511–12.

26 Camann W, Denney R, Holby E, Datta S. A comparison of intrathecal, epidural and intravenous sufentanil for labor analgesia. *Anesthesiology* 1992;**77**:884–7.

27 Heytens L, Cammu H, Camu F. Extradural analgesia during labour using alfentanil. *Br J Anaesth* 1987;**59**:331–7.

28 Bader AM, Ray N, Datta S. Continuous epidural infusion of alfentanil and bupivacaine for labor and delivery. *Int J Obstet Anesth* 1992;**1**:187–90.

29 McGrady EM, Brownhill DK, Davis AG. Epidural diamorphine and bupivacaine in labour. *Anaesthesia* 1989;**44**:400–3.

30 Kestin I, Madden A, Mulvein J, Goodman N. Analgesia for labour and delivery using incremental diamorphine and bupivacaine via a 32-gauge intrathecal catheter. *Br J Anaesth* 1992;**68**:244–7.

31 Sneyd J, Meyer Witting M. Intrathecal diamorphine for obstetric analgesia. *Int J Obstet Anesth* 1992;**1**:153–5.

32 Husemeyer RP, Cummings AJ, Rosenkiewicz JR, Davenport HT. A study of pethidine kinetics and analgesia in women in labour following intravenous, intramuscular and epidural administration. *Br J Clin Pharmacol* 1982;**13**:171–6.

33 Camann WR, Bader AM. Spinal anesthesia for cesarean delivery with meperidine as the sole agent. *Int J Obstet Anesth* 1992;**1**:156–8.

34 Hunt C, Naulty J, Malinow A, Datta S, Ostheimer GW. Epidural butorphanol–bupivacaine for analgesia during labor and delivery. *Anesth Analg* 1989;**68**:323–7.
35 Hatjis C, Meis P. Sinusoidal fetal heart rate pattern associated with butorphanol administration. *Obstet Gynecol* 1986;**67**:377–80.
36 Abboud TK, Shnider SM, Dailey PA *et al*. Intrathecal administration of hyperbaric morphine for the relief of pain in labour. *Br J Anaesth* 1984;**56**:1351–60.
37 Eisenach J, Detweiler D, Hood D. Hemodynamic and analgesic actions of epidurally administered clonidine. *Anesthesiology* 1993;**78**:277–87.
38 Yarnell RW, Ewing DA, Tierney E, Sacralization of epidural block with repeated doses of 0·25% bupivacaine during labor. *Reg Anesth* 1990;**15**:275–9.
39 O'Meara ME, Gin T. Comparison of 0·125% bupivacaine with 0.125% bupivacaine and clonidine as extradural analgesia in the first stage of labour. *Br J Anaesth* 1993;**71**:651–6.
40 Eisenach JC, D'Angelo R, Taylor C, Hood DD. An isobolographic study of epidural clonidine and fentanyl after cesarean section. *Anesth Analg* 1994;**79**:285–90.
41 Brichant JF, Bonhomme V, Mikulski M, Lamy M, Hans P. Admixture of clonidine to extradural bupivacaine for analgesia during labor: effect of varying clonidine doses. *Anesthesiology* 1994;**81**:A1136.
42 Celleno D, Capogna G, Costantino P, Zangrillo A. Comparison of fentanyl with clonidine as adjuvants for epidural analgesia with 0·125% bupivacaine in the first stage of labor. *Int J Obstet Anesth* 1995;**4**:26–9.
43 Chassard D, Mathon L, Dailler F, Golfier F, Tournade JP, Bouletreau. Extradural clonidine combined with sufentanil and 0·0625% bupivacaine for analgesia in labour. *Br J Anaesth* 1996;**77**:458–62.
44 Hood DD, Eisenach JC, Mallak K, Tuttle R. Interaction between intrathecal neostigmine and epidural clonidine in humans. (Abstract) Society for Obstetric Anesthesia and Perinatology, meeting 1995:p44.

8: Indications and contraindications

Indications
  Maternal
    Pain relief
    Hypertensive disease
    Pre-existing disease
    Suspected difficult intubation
  Fetal
    Prematurity
    Breech
    Multiple pregnancy
    Intrauterine death
  Labour
    Prolonged labour
    Trial of labour
    Previous caesarean section
    Instrumental delivery
    Operative management of the third stage
Contraindications
  Maternal refusal
  Coagulation disorders
  Local or systemic sepsis
  Hypovolaemia
  Lack of trained staff
  Allergies

Indications

Regional analgesia may be indicated for the mother, for the baby or for labour itself.

Maternal indications

Effective pain relief

The most common indication for regional analgesia in labour is maternal request. Almost all women find labour painful and among primipara, those experiencing prolonged labours and induced labours the demand for regional analgesia is increased (see below).[1]

Hypertensive disorders of pregnancy

In the absence of coagulopathy, which contraindicates regional techniques, epidural analgesia may be valuable in the management of the pre-eclamptic patient. Sympathetic blockade is not appropriate for the treatment of hypertension in the absence of pain, indeed its effect is only transient and may be associated with impaired placental perfusion. However effective analgesia prevents further surges in blood pressure during painful uterine contractions and, provided cardiac output is maintained and aorto-caval compression avoided, placental perfusion is maintained and may be improved.[2] The catecholamine surge with pain which exacerbates the adverse effects of pre-eclampsia is also inhibited by regional blockade.[3] Instrumental and operative deliveries are often indicated in hypertensive disease and extension of established epidural blockade is probably the ideal method of providing the necessary anaesthesia. Spinal anaesthesia is not ideal since it may lead to a rapid onset of hypotension. Administration of vasopressors, whether prophylactic or therapeutic, is not ideal in pre-eclampsia, where there is increased sensitivity to sympathomimetic amines. Though general anaesthesia is often used, there is an increased possibility of difficulties with intubation, and the danger of surges in blood pressure and the increased morbidity and mortality associated with general anaesthesia should be borne in mind.[4]

Pre-existing disease

Cardiovascular Although the incidence of rheumatic heart disease is decreasing, the number of women with *congenital heart disease* reaching childbearing age is increasing. Congenital heart disease may be classified as left-to-right and right-to-left shunt, and congenital valvular and vascular lesions.[5] Patients with right-to-left shunts, such as Tetralogy of Fallot and Eisenmenger's Syndrome, tolerate pregnancy poorly and have a significant risk of mortality during labour and the puerperium.[6] Death may result from sudden blood loss, increased pulmonary vascular resistance or a fall in systemic vascular resistance.[7] The ability of epidural analgesia to protect a mother from the adverse effects of a stressful labour may nevertheless be of particular value in heart disease. Caution must be exercised, however, as widespread sympathetic block of rapid onset may lead to a dramatic fall in cardiac output. Intravenous fluid must be carefully titrated, with the assistance of invasive monitoring, to prevent either a fall in venous return or overload. Death has been reported following epidural anaesthesia, given by a single large bolus, in the presence of aortic valve disease.[8] Local anaesthetics should be administered slowly and in low dose, possibly with supplemental opioids, whilst aorto-caval compression must be avoided. In the presence of shunt, peripheral vasodilatation may be disastrous as it will exacerbate a right-to-left shunt and may reverse a left-to-right shunt with consequent fall in oxygen saturation.[6]

Primary pulmonary hypertension is most commonly seen in women of childbearing age and, like Eisenmenger's Syndrome, it carries a significant mortality in the peripartum period.[9] Regional analgesia has been successfully used, but the technique must be meticulous, as peripheral vasodilatation with decreased venous return is poorly tolerated.

Respiratory **Asthma** is the most common respiratory disease seen in pregnancy. Bronchospasm may be triggered by the stress and hyperventilation associated with painful labour and regional analgesia may be indicated to reduce this possibility. It is also clearly desirable to avoid the need for general anaesthesia in the asthmatic patient.

Cystic fibrosis is an inherited disorder affecting exocrine glands resulting in malabsorption and respiratory complications. Airflow obstruction from failure to clear secretions leads to recurrent infection and bronchiectasis. Colonisation of the respiratory tract with *Staphylococcus aureus* or pseudomonas is common and predisposes to further infection. Improvements in medical management have resulted in more women surviving to childbearing age. Women with cystic fibrosis are less able to meet the increased respiratory demands of labour and effective analgesia is advantageous. Epidural analgesia is therefore indicated, but must be carefully titrated so that the block does not rise above T8 and interfere with respiratory function.[10] Epidural infusions of low dose bupivacaine with opioids (see Chapter 10) may be particularly useful as motor block is minimised and the upper level of the block is more easily controlled.

Neurological Regional analgesia is useful in the **epileptic** parturient. Hyperventilation produces hypocarbia and may precipitate fitting, whilst the pethidine metabolite norpethidine has convulsant properties. It may also be wise to reduce violent expulsive efforts associated with an uncontrolled bearing down reflex. Regional analgesia has also been recommended for parturients with **myasthenia gravis**[11] in whom it is certainly desirable to avoid the need for general anaesthesia. Any condition in which **increased intracranial pressure** would be dangerous is best managed with regional analgesia although a large volume must not be injected rapidly into the epidural space as this increases intracranial pressure and may precipitate seizures. If raised intracranial pressure is present dural puncture must also be avoided for fear of coning.

Other **Diabetes mellitus** may be best managed with regional analgesia to avoid stress with associated maternal and fetal acidosis, and because instrumental and operative delivery are more commonly needed. The signs of hypoglycaemia may be obscured by epidural analgesia and therefore blood sugar must be closely monitored, especially after delivery, when insulin requirements fall rapidly.

The **obese** obstetric patient poses many anaesthetic problems. General anaesthesia is especially hazardous[8] as airway management may be difficult and oxygen desaturation develops rapidly during induction of general anaesthesia. Hiatus hernia is also more common, increasing the possibility for reflux of stomach contents. Epidural and spinal analgesia may be technically difficult and should therefore be performed early in labour with a cooperative mother. There is a major danger of supine hypotension in the obese parturient, so every precaution must be taken. Every effort should be made to minimise aorto-caval compression, a generous circulatory preload should be given and the anaesthetist should be ready to use vasopressors, calculating the dose carefully on a mg/kg basis.

Regional analgesia is desirable in mothers with **sickle cell anaemia** as it minimises maternal metabolic acidosis and avoids the maternal oxygen desaturation that is associated with inhalational and narcotic analgesia.[12,13] Epidural opioids, however, should be avoided as they may also increase the incidence of maternal desaturation.[14,15]

Suspected difficult intubation

Difficult or failed tracheal intubation during general anaesthesia leading to hypoxia or aspiration of stomach contents is the most common cause of anaesthetic morbidity and mortality in obstetric practice. Any parturient in whom intubation is expected to be difficult and obstetric intervention is thought to be likely should be advised to have regional analgesia.[16,17]

Fetal indications

Prematurity and intrauterine growth retardation

Regional analgesia can produce a significant increase in placental blood flow providing hypotension and aorto-caval compression are avoided.[2,18] Epidural analgesia is particularly useful when forceps or ventouse are used as pelvic floor relaxation allows a less traumatic and more controlled delivery of the fetal head. Indeed, a significant reduction in neonatal mortality and morbidity amongst low birthweight infants has been reported in those whose mothers received epidural analgesia in labour.[19,20]

Breech presentation

Vaginal breech delivery is becoming less common, but in the past the choice of analgesia has been the subject of much debate. Most would consider that controlled delivery of the aftercoming head with a cooperative mother is desirable,[21] although there are those who believe that regional analgesia prevents mothers from pushing effectively. However the evidence for this is not based on randomised trials, and with an increase in caesarean delivery for breech presentation such studies are now unlikely to be performed.

Multiple pregnancy

Multiple pregnancy increases the risks of pre-eclampsia, prematurity and intrauterine growth retardation, each of which may merit regional analgesia in their own right. At delivery the welfare of the second twin is always a matter of concern and effective analgesia allows confirmation of the presenting part and internal version if necessary. If instrumental or operative delivery is required this can proceed without the need for urgent general anaesthesia. Epidural analgesia has also been demonstrated to lessen the deterioration in the acid–base balance of the second twin should there be delay in delivery.[22]

Intrauterine death

Large doses of systemic opioids are often administered in labour following an intrauterine death because it is thought analgesia may be improved and adverse effects on the baby are not an issue. Pain relief is, however, often far from satisfactory whilst side effects such as nausea and vomiting may be severe. Regional analgesia may be preferred for the distressing experience of labour with a known intrauterine death. Moreover epidural analgesia may actually shorten labour in these patients.[23] Prolonged intrauterine death may, however, lead to coagulopathy which must be excluded before instituting a block. With improved antenatal screening, the incidence of mid-trimester termination of pregnancy for fetal abnormality is increasing. Regional analgesia should be considered for these women as induction of labour may be prolonged and painful and, moreover, some form of anaesthesia is frequently required as it is often necessary to evacuate a retained placenta.

Labour indications

Prolonged labour

Prolonged labour can lead to loss of maternal morale and deterioration in fetal acid–base status. Regional analgesia not only helps the mother to regain control and allows her to rest before the exertions of the second stage but also lessens the degree of fetal acidosis.[24,25]

141

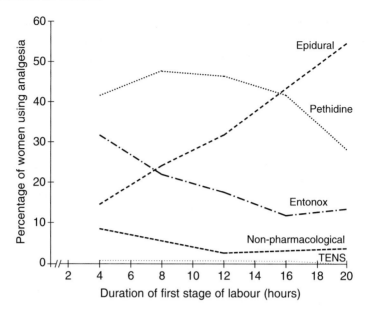

FIGURE 8.1—*Percentage of nulliparous women using each type of pain relief as the dominant method, depending on the duration of labour. Note: those conducting the survey regarded pethidine as dominant over Entonox, despite the inferior analgesic properties of the former. Contrast with Figure 1.1, which includes all types of analgesia used by an individual parturient. (After Chamberlain* et al. (the NBT survey)[1] by permission of the authors and publisher)*

Epidural analgesia is requested more frequently when labour is prolonged (Figure 8.1) and also when induced or augmented with oxytocin,[1] as pain may be particularly severe and prolonged. It has also been suggested that epidural analgesia may increase the rate of cervical dilatation in those with incoordinate uterine action[26] (see also Chapter 9).

Trial of labour

If, for any reason, it is thought likely that caesarean section may be necessary during labour, there is much to be said for establishing epidural analgesia early. First, extending epidural analgesia to provide anaesthesia for surgery is relatively quick and certainly the safest approach. Secondly, to labour in pain and then to require caesarean section can be most demoralising. Regional anaesthesia is now accepted as the safer option for caesarean section. General anaesthesia carries the risks of difficult or failed intubation, aspiration of stomach contents, unplanned awareness, increased blood loss and an increase in deep vein thrombosis when compared to regional techniques.[27] The information from the Confidential Enquiries into

Maternal Deaths suggests that mortality is increased with general anaesthesia and therefore, wherever possible, regional anaesthesia should be encouraged both for elective and emergency caesarean section.

Previous caesarean section

The possibility that regional analgesia may mask the pain of scar dehiscence is no longer accepted as a contraindication to its use after previous caesarean section. Pain is not invariably a feature of scar rupture,[28] while if it occurs it may not be distinguishable by the mother from contraction pain.[29] It is felt in the same area and may initially be felt only during contractions. Other signs such as fetal heart rate abnormalities and blood stained liquor may be more useful in making the diagnosis. Moreover scar pain, when it does occur, is not necessarily concealed by epidural blockade. Crawford first described an epidural sieve in which labour pain but not scar pain was relieved by regional analgesia using low dose local anaesthetics. This may be explained by the fact that labour pain is transmitted largely by Aδ fibres whilst scar pain has a greater C fibre component. Local anaesthetics which block Aδ fibres at lower dose than they do C fibres can therefore in low dose relieve normal contraction pain while blocking the pain originating from a uterine scar less readily. Spinal opioids readily block C fibres and cases have been reported in which the pain of scar rupture has been obtunded following epidural fentanyl.[30-32] Others, however, have described situations where scar pain has persisted despite repeated doses of epidural fentanyl, but nevertheless signs of scar dehiscence were ignored.[33] It is possible that low dose regional analgesia of any type may be helpful in making the diagnosis of scar rupture.[34] If abdominal pain develops in a woman with two warm, dry feet and a block to at least T10, dehiscence should be suspected (see Chapter 12).

Instrumental delivery

The debate surrounding the relationship between regional analgesia and instrumental deliveries continues. One aim of an obstetric anaesthesia service is to provide effective regional blockade for all mothers who are at risk of needing instrumental delivery. Hence it should be regarded as a failure of such a system if a woman without a working block requires obstetric intervention. Epidural analgesia that has been maintained during the second stage may be topped up to provide a painless instrumental delivery. The practice of allowing analgesia to wear off at the end of labour is undesirable. It does not increase the number of spontaneous deliveries[35] and should delivery need to be expedited, analgesia may be inadequate leading to maternal distress and dissatisfaction.[36] A further discussion of management of the second stage appears in Chapter 9 under Instrumental delivery and in Chapter 11. Should there be a need for instrumental delivery in a woman without regional analgesia, spinal anaesthesia is indicated, as rapid pain relief can be achieved.

Operative management of the third stage

In the absence of significant postpartum haemorrhage, regional anaesthesia may be used for the removal of a retained placenta. If an epidural catheter is in place the block may be extended, otherwise spinal anaesthesia may be used. Care must be taken to assess blood loss accurately, as regional anaesthesia may cause profound hypotension in the presence of hypovolaemia. In such circumstances general anaesthesia is preferred unless contraindicated for some other reason.

Contraindications

Maternal refusal

Informed maternal consent must be obtained before regional analgesia, as for any medical procedure or intervention. In early labour details of the technique and effects on mother and baby may be explained between contractions. In advanced labour, however, this may be inappropriate if the mother is severely distressed and suffering mental clouding from other forms of pain relief. It is therefore important to make every effort to explain the techniques involved in regional analgesia and anaesthesia during pregnancy. If a mother refuses to give consent, she should be asked why, in case her fears are unfounded. Reassurance may then lead to consent, when the technique may have a positive benefit. It is surprising that mothers rarely refuse consent for the more hazardous general anaesthesia (see also Chapter 10).

Coagulation disorders[37]

Vascular trauma occurring when inserting an epidural needle or catheter in the presence of abnormal coagulation may result in an expanding spinal haematoma. This may produce cord compression, ischaemia and ultimately neuronal death and thus immediate surgical decompression is required. Although this complication is well recognised in older sick patients on full anticoagulation, case reports involving parturients are rare.[38,39] In one large retrospective survey of half a million parturients only a single case is to be found[40] while *none* appears in other surveys. Nevertheless, it is such a grave complication that regional techniques are contraindicated when bleeding disorders are present. Coagulopathy may pre-exist or may develop during pregnancy, taking the form of thrombocytopenia, HELLP syndrome or disseminated intravascular coagulation. Women may require full

144

anticoagulation because of deep vein thrombosis or valvular heart conditions and coagulopathy may develop in several obstetric conditions including pre-eclampsia, placental abruption, intrauterine death and amniotic fluid embolus. Low dose heparin and aspirin are not designed to do more than prevent coagulation within the vascular compartment and evidence has accumulated to suggest that epidural blockade is safe in patients receiving low dose heparin[41] and aspirin.[42]

There is still much debate about when regional techniques should be withheld in a suspected bleeding disorder and no one test reliably indicates their safety. Where there is doubt, a history should be taken of recent drug treatment, previous bleeding troubles, such as may follow dental extraction, or easy bruising, and coexisting medical disease. A platelet count provides useful information. Epidural insertion is usually considered safe when the count is greater than $100 \times 10^9/l$, but below $80 \times 10^9/l$ regional techniques are usually considered contraindicated. Between 80 and $100 \times 10^9/l$ a further test of coagulation should be performed. The platelet count should be compared with previous results as a substantial drop in number may signify imminent bleeding problems. It should also be remembered that the platelet count gives no indication of platelet function and with good function as few as $40 \times 10^9/l$ suffice. Though epidural catheters have from time to time been sited inadvertently in the presence of extremely low platelet counts without mishap,[43] accidental vessel puncture, probably a prerequisite of epidural haematoma, cannot be predicted or avoided with certainty. Where doubt exists as to the safety of regional analgesia the relative advantages and disadvantages must be considered and the catheter inserted with no force.

The bleeding time has been suggested as a simple bedside test to provide an indication of abnormal coagulation. The test tends to be observer-dependent and is not a reliable indicator for the safety of regional analgesia.[44] Thrombelastography has been used widely in cardiac and liver surgery to aid in the treatment of bleeding problems. Its role as a guide to providing regional analgesia in a parturient with suspected coagulopathy remains to be determined.

Local or systemic sepsis

The introduction of infection risks the development of epidural abscess or, if the dura is punctured, meningitis. It is generally accepted that regional analgesia should never be performed through an area of skin sepsis but the risk from blood-borne sepsis is also significant, particularly in the presence of risk factors (see Box), such as prolonged catheterisation and immunocompromise. Failure to administer local anaesthetic solutions may increase risk since they have an antimicrobial effect.[45-47] It should be

145

Aetiology of epidural abscess

- Source of infection
  Epidural needle
  Epidural catheter
  Adjacent skin
  Injectate
  Blood borne

- Risk factors
  Poor aseptic technique
  Prolonged catheterisation
  Absence of antimicrobial local anaesthetic
  Bacteraemia or septicaemia
  Thoracic catheterisation
  Immunocompromise: steroids, diabetes, HIV

emphasised that epidural abscess is frequently reported in the absence of epidural instrumentation,[48–50] though if an epidural catheter is present it will inevitably be blamed.

If regional analgesia is requested in a febrile parturient, the risks of subsequent abscess or meningitis may be reduced by appropriate antibiotic therapy.[51] The risk of withholding regional analgesia, especially where operative delivery is likely, must be balanced against the chances of meningitis or abscess.[52]

The presence of severe backache, local tenderness, pyrexia and leucocytosis should alert one to the possibility of epidural abscess *before* the advent of neurological sequelae as urgent laminectomy is required to prevent permanent neurological damage.[53]

Active herpes simplex type 2 infection requires caution. In primary infection the painful genital lesions are associated with a transient viraemia, whilst in secondary infection a viraemia is usually prevented by maternal antibodies. In the presence of active infection, mothers are delivered by caesarean section. Retrospective studies have suggested regional analgesia during secondary infection is probably safe,[54] but there is little information about primary infection. The anaesthetist must therefore assess the risks and benefits of different techniques in each case.

It has been suggested that epidural morphine may promote reactivation of latent herpes simplex virus,[55] although this has not been demonstrated with intrathecal morphine.[56,57] In view of its other side effects, epidural morphine is best avoided in women with a history of herpes simplex infections.

146

Hypovolaemia

In the presence of hypovolaemia, autonomic blockade with resulting vasodilatation can produce a catastrophic fall in cardiac output, and the ability to compensate for on-going haemorrhage is lost. Caution is essential in situations where hypovolaemia may develop, such as during caesarean section for placenta praevia. If the placenta is anterior, bleeding may be rapid and excessive, but placenta praevia in any position increases the risk of bleeding from large vessels in the lower segment. An anterior placenta praevia in a woman with a uterine scar from previous caesarean section should be seen as an absolute contraindication to regional blockade as the risk of placenta percreta or accreta is high. Here catastrophic haemorrhage is likely.

Lack of trained staff

Although the benefits of regional analgesia can be great, they make heavy demands on staff. Suitably trained anaesthetic staff must be available 24 hours a day with trained midwives monitoring both mother and baby for the duration of regional blockade.[58] Training of both medical and midwifery staff should involve management of the parturient with regional analgesia as well as the side effects and possible complications. If the safety of mother and baby cannot be ensured because of a lack of trained staff, regional analgesia should not be employed.

The request for epidural analgesia by a woman who has opted for midwifery-led care probably necessitates her transfer to full obstetric care. This is because she is not having the quick easy labour that she anticipated, suggesting that low-tech care may not be suitable and the requirement for obstetric intervention is increased.

Allergies

Although not a contraindication to regional analgesia *per se*, a history of anaphylactic reaction to a drug or material requires potential allergens to be avoided. Allergy to ester local anaesthetics is not uncommon. Fortunately amides are less allergenic, although reactions have been reported with lignocaine,[59] prilocaine[60] and bupivacaine.[61] Many patients who believe themselves to be allergic to local anaesthetics have experienced only a faint, an adrenaline reaction in the dental chair or systemic toxicity following accidental intravenous injection.[62] Where doubt exists, intradermal testing may help with the diagnosis, although this carries the risk of a systemic reaction.

An increasingly well-recognised problem is that of latex allergy.[63] Latex is a component of many pieces of anaesthetic equipment such as gloves,

147

drapes, intravenous cannulae and fluids, syringes, and some epidural and spinal packs.

References

1 Chamberlain G, Wraight A, Steer P. *Pain and its relief in childbirth: the results of a survey conducted by the National Childbirth Trust.* Edinburgh: Churchill Livingstone, 1993.
2 Jouppila R, Jouppila P, Hollmen A, Koivula A. Epidural analgesia and placental blood flow during labour in pregnancies complicated by hypertension. *Br J Obstet Gynaecol* 1979;**86**:969–72.
3 Ramanathan J, Coleman P, Sibai B. Anesthetic modification of hemodynamic and neuroendocrine stress responsiveness to cesarean delivery in women with severe preeclampsia. *Anesth Analg* 1991;**73**:772–9.
4 Robson SC. The danger of convulsions precludes the use of regional analgesia for caesarean section in fulminating preeclampsia – Opposer. *Int J Obstet Anesth* 1993;**2**:104–5.
5 Mangano DT. Anesthesia for the pregnant cardiac patient. In: Shnider SM, Levinson G, eds. *Anesthesia for obstetrics.* Baltimore: Williams & Wilkins, 1993;485–523.
6 Stoddart P, O'Sullivan G. Eisenmenger's syndrome in pregnancy: a case report and review. *Int J Obstet Anesth* 1993;**2**:159–68.
7 Gleicher N, Midwall J, Hochberger D, Jaffin H. Eisenmenger's syndrome and pregnancy. *Obstet Gynecol Surv* 1979;**34**:721–41.
8 Department of Health and others. *Report on Confidential Enquiries into Maternal Deaths in the UK, 1988–1990.* London: HMSO, 1994.
9 Khan MJ, Bhatt SB, Krye JJ. Anesthetic considerations for parturients with pulmonary hypertension: review of the literature and clinical presentation. *Int J Obstet Anesth* 1996; **5**:36–42.
10 Howell PR, Kent N, Douglas MJ. Anaesthesia for the parturient with cystic fibrosis. *Int J Obstet Anesth* 1993;**2**:152–8.
11 Rolbin WH, Levinson G, Shnider SM, Wright RG. Anesthetic considerations for myasthenia gravis and pregnancy. *Anesth Analg* 1978;**57**:441–7.
12 Reed PN, Colquhoun AD, Hanning CD. Maternal oxygenation during normal labour. *Br J Anaesth* 1989;**62**:316–18.
13 Deckardt R, Fembacher PM, Scheider KTM, Graeff H. Maternal arterial oxygen saturation during labor and delivery: pain dependent alterations and effects on the newborn. *Obstet Gynecol* 1987;**70**:21–5.
14 Griffin R, Reynolds F. Maternal hypoxaemia during labour and delivery, the influence of analgesia and effect on neonatal outcome. *Anaesthesia* 1995;**50**:151–6.
15 Porter JS, Bonello E, Reynolds F. The effect of epidural opioids on maternal oxygenation during labour and delivery. *Anaesthesia* 1996;**51**:899–903.
16 Wilson ME, Spiegelhalter D, Robertson JA, Lesser P. Predicting difficult intubation. *Br J Anaesth* 1988;**61**:211–16.
17 Rocke DA, Murray WB, Rout CC, Gouws E. Relative risk analysis of factors associated with difficult intubation in obstetric anesthesia. *Anesthesiology* 1992;**77**:67–73.
18 Hollmen A, Jouppila R, Jouppila P, Koivula A, Vierola H. Effect of extradural analgesia using bupivacaine and 2-chloroprocaine on intervillous blood flow during normal labour. *Br J Anaesth* 1982;**54**:837–42.
19 David H, Rosen M. Perinatal mortality after epidural analgesia. *Anaesthesia* 1976;**31**: 1054–9.
20 Osbourne GK, Patel NB, Howat RCL. A comparison of outcome of low birthweight pregnancy in Glasgow and Dundee. *Health Bull (Edinb)* 1984;**42**:68–77.
21 Van Zundert A, Vaes L, Soetens M et al. Are breech deliveries an indication for lumbar epidural analgesia? *Anesth Analg* 1991;**72**:399–403.
22 Crawford JS. A prospective study of 200 consecutive twin deliveries. *Anaesthesia* 1987; **42**:33–43.

148

23 Lurie S, Blickstein L, Feinstein M, Matzkel A, Ezri T, Soroker D. Influence of epidural anaesthesia on the course of labour in patients with antepartum fetal death. *Aust NZ J Obstet Gynaecol* 1991;**31**:227–8.
24 Pearson JF, Davies P. The effect of continuous lumbar epidural analgesia upon fetal acid-base status during the first stage of labour. *J Obstet Gynaecol Br Commonwlth* 1974;**81**: 971–4.
25 Pearson JF, Davies P. The effect of continuous lumbar epidural analgesia upon fetal acid-base status during the second stage of labour. *J Obstet Gynaecol Br Commonwlth* 1974;**81**: 975–9.
26 Moir DD, Willocks J. Management of incoordinate uterine action under continuous epidural analgesia. *BMJ* 1967;**iii**:396.
27 O'Sullivan G. Regional or general anaesthesia for caesarean section. In: Reynolds F, ed. *Epidural and spinal blockade in obstetrics*. London: Baillière Tindall, 1990;127–38.
28 Molloy BG, Sheil O, Duignan NM. Delivery after caesarean section: review of 2176 consecutive cases. *BMJ* 1987;**294**:1645–7.
29 Case BD, Corcoran R, Jeffcote N, Randle GH. Caesarean section and its place in modern obstetric practice. *J Obstet Gynaecol Br Commonwlth* 1971;**78**:203–14.
30 Tehan B. Abolition of the extradural sieve by the addition of fentanyl to extradural bupivacaine. *Br J Anaesth* 1992;**69**:520–1.
31 Rashiq S, Huston LJ. Fentanyl and the extradural sieve. *Br J Anaesth* 1993;**71**:920.
32 McBeth C. Epidural opioids and previous caesarean section. *Int J Obstet Anesth* 1995;**4**: 251–3.
33 Rowbottom SJ, Tabrizian I. Epidural analgesia and uterine rupture during labour. *Anaesth Intens Care* 1994;**22**:79–80.
34 Groves PA, Oriol NE. The extradural sieve. *Br J Anaesth* 1994;**73**:430–431.
35 Phillips KC, Thomas TA. Second stage of labour with or without extradural analgesia. *Anaesthesia* 1983;**38**:972–6.
36 Morgan BM, Bulpitt CJ, Clifton P, Lewis PJ. Analgesia and satisfaction in childbirth (The Queen Charlotte's 1000 Mother Survey). *Lancet* 1982;**ii**:808–10.
37 Vandermeulen EP, Van Aken H, Vermylen J. Anticoagulants and spinal-epidural anesthesia. *Anesth Analg* 1994;**79**:1165–77.
38 Lao TL, Halpern SH, MacDonald D, Huh C. Spinal subdural haematoma in a parturient after attempted epidural anaesthesia. *Can J Anaesth* 1993;**40**:340–45.
39 Brougher RJ, Ramage D. Spinal subdural haematoma following combined spinal epidural anaesthesia. *Anaesth Intens Care* 1995;**23**:111–13.
40 Scott DB, Hibbard BM. Serious non-fatal complications associated with extradural block in obstetric practice. *Br J Anaesth* 1990;**64**:537–41.
41 Letsky EA. Haemostasis and epidural anaesthesia. *Int J Obstet Anesth* 1991;**1**:51–4.
42 Nelson-Piercy C, De Swiet M. The place of low-dose aspirin in pregnancy. *Int J Obstet Anaesth* 1994;**3**:3–6.
43 Hew-Wing P, Rolbin SH, Amato D. Epidural anaesthesia and thrombocytopenia. *Anaesthesia* 1989;**44**:775–7.
44 Rodgers RPC, Levin J. A critical reappraisal of bleeding time. *Semin Thromb Hemost* 1990; **16**:1–20.
45 Schmitt RM, Rosenkranz HS. Antimicrobial activity of local anaesthetics. *Anesthesiology* 1989;**71**:988–90.
46 Borum SE, McLeskey CH, Williamson JB, Harris FS, Knight AB. Epidural abscess after obstetric epidural analgesia. *Anesthesiology* 1995;**82**:1523–6.
47 Ngan Kee WD, Jones MR, Thomas P, Worth RJ. Extradural abscess complicating extradural anaesthesia for caesarean section. *Br J Anaesth* 1992;**69**:647–52.
48 Baker AS, Oemann RG, Swartz MN, Richardson EP. Spinal epidural abscess. *N Engl J Med* 1975;**293**:463–8.
49 Male CG, Martin R. Puerperal spinal epidural abscess. *Lancet* 1973;**i**:608–609.
50 Kitching AJ, Rice ASC. Extradural abscess in the postpartum period. *Br J Anaesth* 1993; **70**:703.
51 Carp H, Bailey S. The association between meningitis and dural puncture in bacteremic rats. *Anesthesiology* 1992;**76**:739–42.

52 Chestnut DH. Spinal anesthesia in the febrile patient. *Anesthesiology* 1992;**76**:667–9.
53 Bromage PR. Spinal epidural abscess: pursuit of vigilance. *Br J Anaesth* 1993;**70**:471–3.
54 Bader AM, Camann WR, Datta S. Anesthesia for cesarean delivery in patients with herpes simplex type-2 infections. *Reg Anesth* 1990;**15**:261–3.
55 Boyle RK. Herpes simplex labialis after epidural or parenteral morphine: a randomized prospective trial in an Australian obstetric population. *Anaesth Intens Care* 1995;**23**:433–7.
56 Norris MC, Weiss J, Carney M, Leighton BL. The incidence of herpes simplex virus labialis after caesarean delivery. *Int J Obstet Anesth* 1994;**3**:127–31.
57 Abouleish EA. Intrathecal morphine as a cause for herpes simplex should be scratched out. *Anesthesiology* 1991;**74**:199.
58 Obstetric Anaesthetists Association. Recommended minimum standards for obstetric anaesthesia services. *Int J Obstet Anesth* 1995;**4**:125–8.
59 Noble DS, Pierce GFM. Allergy to lignocaine. A case history. *Lancet* 1961;**ii**:1436.
60 Yeoman CM. Hypersensitivity to prilocaine. *Br Dent J* 1982;**153**:69–70.
61 Brown DT, Beamish D, Wildsmith JAW. Allergic reaction to an amide local anaesthetic. *Br J Anaesth* 1981;**53**:435–7.
62 Babajews AV, Ivanyi L. The relationship between in vivo and in vitro reactivity of patients with a history of allergy to local anaesthetics. *Br Dent J* 1982;**152**:385–7.
63 Stewart PD, Bogod D. Latex anaphylaxis during late pregnancy. *Int J Obstet Anesth* 1995;**4**:48–50.

9: Effects and complications

Effects of regional blockade on the mother

Sensory block

Block of pain fibres in the lower thoracic and upper lumbar nerve roots prevents the lower abdominal pain of uterine contraction. Perineal pain is relieved by blocking the sacral nerve roots (see Figure 3.2).

Motor block

Motor block during regional anaesthesia is dependent on the cumulative dose of local anaesthetic, thus motor block becomes progressively more

151

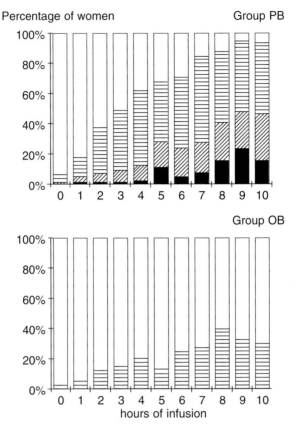

FIGURE 9.1—*Motor block during epidural infusion. PB = 0·125% bupivacaine; OB = 0·0625% bupivacaine with opioid. Motor block: white = grade 0; horizontal shading = grade 1; diagonal shading = grade 2; black = grade 3. (From Russell and Reynolds[2] by permission of the publisher)*

severe with duration of epidural analgesia (Figure 9.1). The possible relationship between motor block and instrumental delivery is discussed later in this chapter.

Maternal satisfaction with regional analgesia is reduced as motor block increases. Allowing a reduction in dose of local anaesthetic by adding opioids to the epidural solution whether given by bolus[1] or infusion[2] therefore increases maternal satisfaction. A comparison of combined spinal–epidural analgesia, where motor block is so minimal that mothers may ambulate, with traditional epidural top-ups has again demonstrated an increase in maternal satisfaction with analgesia.[3] Effective analgesia *per se* does not ensure that childbirth is a rewarding experience. Other factors are as important.[4]

Regional analgesia for labour should not involve a motor block high enough to cause a deterioration in respiratory function.

Autonomic block

Local anaesthetics readily block conduction in preganglionic autonomic B fibres in low doses. This produces vasodilatation and decreased sweating. Indeed, the presence of two warm, dry feet is a useful objective test of an effective bilateral block. Vasodilatation may lead to venous pooling in the lower half of the body and thus increases the likelihood of maternal hypotension and reduced placental perfusion. This is exacerbated by the supine position (see Chapter 7, Aorto-caval compression, p. 125–6). Other aspects of autonomic blockade are described in Chapter 7 (see pages 125–127).

Proprioception

Dorsal column function is progressively impaired by increasing doses of epidural and spinal local anaesthetics. Such impairment may render ambulation in mothers receiving regional analgesia unsafe. Buggy and colleagues demonstrated that following 30 mg of epidural bupivacaine 66% of women developed abnormal distal proprioception.[5] Such impairment was, however, found in less than 10% of mothers who received an intrathecal injection of 2·5 mg bupivacaine with 25 µg fentanyl as part of a combined spinal–epidural technique[6] (see Chapter 10).

Maternal temperature

Epidural analgesia in labour is associated with a rise in maternal temperature.[7,8] The temperature of parturients receiving epidural analgesia has been shown to rise by 1°C over 7 hours[7] and to rise significantly higher than with systemic medication,[8] though without apparent effect on either mother or baby. The mechanism for the temperature rise remains uncertain, but high ambient temperature in delivery rooms combined with decreased sweating and a lack of hyperventilation have been postulated.

Stress response

Stress may be caused by fear of hospitals, anxiety about labour outcome, mistrust of carers and starvation in the face of extra metabolic demands. The pain of labour is, however, the overriding cause of stress, and in the majority of parturients this remains even in the absence of anxiety or fear. The physiological and hormonal changes that make up the stress response[9] are designed to maintain cerebral and myocardial perfusion, but in labour there is an unwanted reduction in visceral, including placental, blood flow[10] and adverse biochemical changes.

The stress response involves the hypothalamic/pituitary axis with release of ACTH and β lipotropin which are cleaved from the parent molecule pro-opiomelanocortin. These in turn cause increases in cortisol and β endorphin levels, though the latter unfortunately appears unable to attenuate labour pain in the majority of sufferers. Activation of the sympathoadrenal system also causes catecholamine release. The metabolic outcome of the increased cortisol and catecholamine levels is hyperglycaemia with poor insulin response, lipolysis with release of free fatty acids and an increase in ketone and lactate levels. High catecholamine levels have potentially adverse effects on β receptors, reducing uterine contractility, and on α receptors, reducing placental blood flow.

Many studies have demonstrated that effective analgesia can attenuate these adverse effects. Westgren and colleagues observed that epidural analgesia with bupivacaine top-ups attenuates the rise in maternal plasma ACTH and cortisol with no significant change in glucose or catecholamines[11] while a more accurate assay system demonstrated significant reduction in

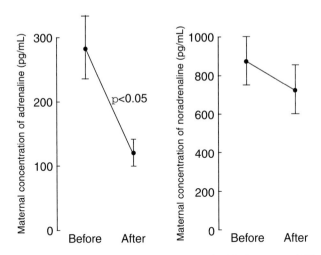

FIGURE 9.2—*Catecholamine concentrations (mean ± SEM) in maternal blood sampled before and after epidural analgesia in labour: left, adrenaline; right, noradrenaline (From data of Shnider et al[12])*

catecholamines[12] (Figure 9.2). Fortunately, the neonatal stress response, important for adaptation to extrauterine life, is maintained in the presence of maternal epidural analgesia. The reduction in maternal plasma adrenaline together with blockade of neurogenic uterine vasoconstriction explains the improvement in intervillous blood flow following epidural analgesia,[13] particularly in those with pre-eclampsia,[14,15] and the reduction in fetal and neonatal acidosis which is otherwise exacerbated by stress.

Bladder function

Difficulty passing urine is not uncommon during labour. Regional analgesia with both local anaesthetic and opioids increases the incidence of urinary retention. With a working epidural the desire to void may not be present although a full bladder may cause low abdominal pain. Spinal opioids produce retention by inhibiting sacral parasympathetic outflow resulting in relaxation of the detrusor muscle.[16,17] Although women receiving epidural opioids may have difficulty voiding, with perseverance they are usually able to pass urine spontaneously. Labouring women should be encouraged to pass urine regularly, especially if they are receiving regional analgesia. If they are unable to pass urine, the bladder should be emptied with a catheter to prevent distension which may lead to postnatal urinary dysfunction.

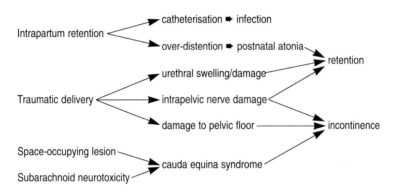

FIGURE 9.3—*Causes of postpartum bladder disturbance. (From Russell and Reynolds*[18] *by permission of the publishers)*

Postnatal urinary disorders have many possible causes (Figure 9.3) and may occur after vaginal delivery in which regional analgesia has not been used.[19] Difficult delivery resulting in haematoma, or urethral swelling, may lead to urinary retention, whereas perineal trauma or pelvic nerve damage may produce incontinence.

Dural puncture

The clinical picture and outcome depend on whether the dura is punctured deliberately by a fine atraumatic spinal needle or unintentionally during the search for the epidural space using a large epidural needle. With correct teaching unintentional dural puncture should occur in less than 1% of cases.

An epidural needle may pass through both the dura and arachnoid, resulting in the free flow of CSF. Alternatively, the dura may be torn by the needle leaving the arachnoid intact. Here the catheter may pass into either the epidural or subdural space or pierce the delicate arachnoid to lie intrathecally.

When fluid leaks from needle or catheter, a persistent or rapid flow strongly suggests CSF. If there is doubt whether the fluid is saline, CSF or local anaesthetic, its temperature, pH and sugar content may be tested. These act only as a guide and are not 100% reliable[20] and therefore a test dose (see Chapter 10) should be administered before the main dose. If the fluid is definitely CSF, opinion is divided regarding further management. Some prefer to introduce a catheter into the CSF, if this has not already been done, and continue with spinal analgesia. Others remove the needle or catheter and resite the epidural at a higher interspace. The disadvantages of this popular policy are that analgesia is delayed, there is a risk of a second dural puncture and there is an increased risk of unexpected high block[21] and even total spinal anaesthesia. Furthermore, extension of the block for caesarean section is contraindicated and *de novo* spinal anaesthesia dangerous,[22] leaving general anaesthesia the only option. With a spinal catheter, effective analgesia for labour can be provided without delay, and the block may be rapidly extended should caesarean section be required. Catheters lying subdurally should be removed as there is significant risk of arachnoid rupture and total spinal anaesthesia (see below).

Accidental total spinal

As the dose requirement for epidural analgesia is ten-fold greater than that for spinal use, unrecognised injection into the CSF of an epidural dose of local anaesthetic results in accidental total spinal anaesthesia. The block rapidly extends in a cephalad direction causing severe hypotension, respiratory failure, unconsciousness and death if treatment is not started immediately. The mother requires intubation, ventilation and circulatory support until the effects of the local anaesthetic have worn off. Hypotension must be treated with intravenous fluids, vasopressors and left uterine displacement. Urgent delivery of the baby may be required to overcome aorto-caval compression and so permit resuscitation.

An epidural dose of opioid given intrathecally produces excessive somnolence and respiratory depression which is less disastrous and may be overcome by intravenous naloxone. However, the effects of naloxone may be shorter-lasting than those of the spinal opioid and repeated doses may be required.

Headache

Puncture of the dura, whether deliberate or unintentional, may lead to a CSF leak and a low pressure headache. The incidence and severity of headache are related to the size, design and bevel direction of the needle. Up to 75% of mothers develop headache if a 16 or 18 gauge needle, such as an epidural needle, has been used. Spinal needles (see below) are of smaller gauge and thus produce fewer, less severe headaches. The design of the needle point is also related to the incidence of headache. Cutting (Quincke) points of 26 gauge produce headache in 5–25% of mothers whereas finer 29 gauge needles produce few headaches but are technically difficult to use.[23,24] A needle with an atraumatic point (Whitacre, Sprotte) is associated with fewer headaches than cutting needles of similar size and is therefore the needle of choice in obstetric patients. Headache is also less likely if the bevel of a Quincke or a Tuohy needle is kept parallel to the long axis of the spine. Such a technique necessitates rotating the epidural needle within the epidural space, which itself increases the likelihood of tearing the dura[25] and is not recommended.

To reduce the incidence of headache it has been stated that excessive bearing down in the second stage should be avoided. However, the elective use of forceps has not been associated with a reduction in the incidence of headaches.[26] It would therefore seem reasonable to allow the mother to push for a short time if spontaneous delivery appears likely. Diagnosis and management of dural puncture headache are discussed in Chapter 12.

Local anaesthetic toxicity

Systemic toxic effects of local anaesthetics are described in Chapter 7.

Toxic reactions may occur from accidental intravenous injection, or following overdose, whether acute or cumulative. Since the advent of bupivacaine, with its reduced rate of absorption into the circulation, toxicity from overdose has been much less of a problem than with older drugs such as lignocaine. There are two situations in which systemic toxicity may occur. The first is when an epidural catheter is inadvertently placed intravascularly. This is almost certainly the cause of the bupivacaine-related deaths seen in the USA, where the use of small single hole catheters may have made intravascular placement difficult to detect. Use of three-holed catheters improves the likelihood of detecting intravascular placement, although too strong aspiration may still produce false-negative results. It is therefore imperative to maintain both visual and verbal contact with the mother when administering any epidural bolus to detect early signs of local anaesthetic toxicity, such as light-headedness and circumoral tingling.

The other situation in which systemic toxicity has been reported is following large epidural doses of bupivacaine for caesarean section, when women have received well in excess of the manufacturer's recommended maximum (see Table 9.1). In the two cases reported by Thorburn and

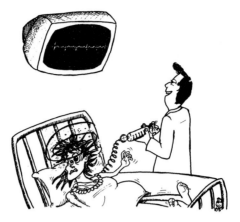

"Now don't you fret, Mrs Firkin, my eyes are glued to your ECG."

TABLE 9.1—*Data from case reports of patients with symptomatic bupivacaine toxicity*

Caesarean section	Bupivacaine con. (%)	Total dose (mg)	Time period	Dose (mg/kg)	Toxic symptoms
Emergency	0·375 0·5	357·5	10 h	4·9	convulsions
Emergency	0·35 0·5	356·25	9 h	6·48	convulsions
Elective	0·5	300	3 h 7 min	4·47	convulsions
Elective	0·75	382·5	1 h 58 min	5·97	convulsions (plasma conc. 2·5 µg/ml)
Elective	0·75	225	48 min	2·71	drowsiness
Elective	0·5	90	8 min	1·32	convulsions (probably eclamptic)
Elective	0·75 0·75	525	60 min	7·09	slurred speech, confusion

Data from Thorburn and Moir[27] and Crawford *et al.*[28]

Moir, both mothers had received prolonged administration in labour and a total dose over 350 mg of bupivacaine.[27] Convulsions have also been reported after epidural analgesia for elective caesarean section when large doses of 0·5% bupivacaine were needed to establish the block because of an excessively slow incremental dose regimen.[28] Nevertheless Laishley *et al*[29] gave 100 mg bolus doses of bupivacaine to 40 women who had received up to 328 mg for labour analgesia. All blocks were satisfactory, whether or not adrenaline was used. No women had toxic plasma levels of bupivacaine or exhibited signs of systemic toxicity.

158

Neurological sequelae

Transient postpartum neurological symptoms have been reported after approximately 1 in 530 deliveries.[30] An increased frequency was observed in those who received general or regional anaesthesia, perhaps because difficult labours in which the need for regional analgesia was greater were also those more likely to produce neurological symptoms. Neurological problems are more commonly due to labour itself than to regional block-ade,[31] although postpartum problems are almost invariably attributed to regional analgesia. In one survey Holdcroft and colleagues reported neurological sequelae with a postpartum frequency of about 1 in 2500 deliveries but epidural analgesia was associated with prolonged dysfunction in only 1 in 13 000 deliveries.[32] A retrospective UK survey reported neurological symptoms after regional analgesia with a frequency of 1 in 4700[33] and a more recent prospective survey, 1 in 1000.[34] Neither study, however, contained data from a control group in which regional analgesia had not been used.

TABLE 9.2—*Mechanisms for neurological complications after regional analgesia*

Paraplegia and cauda equina syndrome	
Space-occupying lesions	Haematoma
	Abscess
Neurotoxicity and	Inappropriate solution
arachnoiditis	Detergents
	Antiseptics
Ischaemia	Hypotension/anterior spinal artery syndrome
Nerve root lesions	Trauma
	Compression
Peripheral lesions	Neglected nerve compression
Cranial nerve palsy	CSF leak
Cranial subdural haematoma	CSF leak
Coning	CSF leak

Mechanisms of neurological complications after regional analgesia (Table 9.2)

Paraplegia and cauda equina syndromes

(1) *Space-occupying lesion* A space-occupying lesion within the confines of the vertebral canal can cause paraplegia, cauda equina syndrome or nerve root lesions by compression of the spinal cord, cauda equina or isolated nerves or their blood supply. Such compression may arise from spinal haematoma or abscess. Haematoma is extremely rare in the obstetric population, but abscess is of greater concern (see Chapter 8, Contraindications).

(2) *Neurotoxicity* Neurotoxicity within the epidural space is difficult to achieve, but has been reported following injection of hypertonic potassium chloride[35] and the use of preservative-containing solutions from multi-dose vials[36] causing paraplegia. A large variety of drugs have been injected both

159

deliberately and inadvertently into the epidural space, producing little other than systemic effect and reversible neural blockade.[37] The same is not true for the subarachnoid space, where nerve roots are vulnerable to neurolysis, while irritant solutions may cause arachnoiditis. The result may be radicular irritation or permanent damage, typically causing cauda equina syndrome. Neurological problems have been reported following either intended[38-43] or accidental spinal injection.[44-47] The use of microspinal catheters has fallen into disrepute following several cases of cauda equina syndrome.[41] In these cases pooling of hyperbaric 5% lignocaine was thought to be the cause of sacral nerve damage. More recently, more dilute solutions of intrathecal lignocaine have been reported to produce transient neurological symptoms.[43] Such problems have not been observed with bupivacaine. Chemical contamination of reusable spinal needles by detergents has in the past been implicated in arachnoiditis.[48] More recently, chemical meningitis following combined spinal epidural analgesia has been attributed to iodine-containing skin preparation solutions.[49]

(3) *Ischaemia* Ischaemic damage of the spinal cord may follow profound and prolonged hypotension. However this situation is most unlikely in obstetric practice, where every effort is made to avoid a reduction in blood pressure which may compromise placental perfusion and fetal well-being. However, cases have been reported in which an anterior spinal artery syndrome has been suspected as a cause of postnatal neurological dysfunction.[33,50,51]

Nerve root lesions Nerve root trauma may be caused by either needle or catheter if they stray from the midline. Transient paraesthesia often occurs during catheter insertion, suggesting that the catheter has touched a sensory nerve root. Trauma to a nerve root causes pain in the appropriate dermatome and may occasionally lead to paraesthesia lasting several weeks. More prolonged neurological dysfunction has been reported following epidural analgesia using a styletted catheter.[52] Damage to nerve roots during spinal analgesia also occurs and symptoms may be more protracted and severe than with catheter damage.

Peripheral lesions If a mother lies in one position for a long time, in the presence of regional analgesia, symptoms of pressure on peripheral nerves may go unrecognised because resulting numbness and motor block may be attributed to epidural blockade.[53] Immobility resulting from epidural analgesia has also been reported to cause pressure sores over the ischial tuberosities or heels.[21]

Neurological complications in the absence of regional analgesia
There is a tendency for clinicians to attribute all postnatal neurological symptoms to regional anaesthesia. It has, however, been demonstrated that

160

such problems are four to six times more likely to have an obstetric rather than anaesthetic cause.[31,32] Obstetric entrapment neuropathies can affect the lumbosacral plexus, the femoral and obturator nerves and, more commonly, the lateral cutaneous nerve of the thigh. Fetal malposition, cephalopelvic disproportion, incorrect placement in the lithotomy position and difficult vaginal delivery all increase the risk. The overall occurrence of such compressive neuropathies is, however, declining with the increase in the caesarean section rate.

It should always be borne in mind that neurological disorders may arise spontaneously in the peripartum period, thus in any case of neurological dysfunction after childbirth, it is essential to demonstrate the mechanism whereby the damage occurred. The mother should be referred promptly to a neurologist or neurosurgeon who can identify the site of the lesion accurately and impartially and determine the appropriate investigations and management. In the case of a space-occupying lesion, early surgical intervention may be essential to preserve function.

Backache

Local tenderness at the site of needle insertion is common in the first few days after delivery. It follows epidural analgesia in approximately 35–45% of women,[2,54] and spinals in 10–30%[24,55] – the incidence being related to needle size and ease of insertion. More generalised short-term backache is reported by up to 20% of those women who receive regional analgesia in labour and also in 40% of those who use other methods of pain relief.[19]

Long-term backache was found to be associated with epidural analgesia in labour in two large retrospective studies.[56,57] In both, the incidence of new backache in those receiving epidurals was approximately 18% compared to 11% in those who did not. In these two studies, however, antenatal backache was reported by only 9% and 25%, whereas prospective studies demonstrated that 50% of women suffer with backache during pregnancy, often continuing into the postnatal period, the discrepancy reflecting inaccurate recall. In prospective studies with more accurate documentation of antenatal backache,[58–60] long-term backache has been no more common after epidural analgesia than after other forms of pain relief. The only predictive factor for long-term backache is probably the presence of antenatal backache, and neither incidence nor severity of motor block appears to be significant.[58]

Gastrointestinal function

Gastric emptying is delayed during labour, and it may be further reduced by the administration of parenteral opioids.[61] This increases the risk of

161

maternal aspiration should urgent general anaesthesia be required. Epidural local anaesthetics do not delay gastric emptying, though bolus doses of opioids given by the epidural route may do so.[62] Continuous epidural infusion of low dose bupivacaine with fentanyl appears not to affect stomach emptying[63] (see Chapter 6).

Effects of regional blockade on labour and delivery

There is still much debate about the effects of regional analgesia on the progress and outcome of labour. There is certainly an association between the use of regional analgesia and the length of both the first and second stages of labour and the need for instrumental delivery. The key issue is whether this represents a causal relationship. Many workers have investigated this subject but unfortunately most studies have been flawed by either methodological problems or dubious interpretation of results. Unrandomised studies are frequently quoted but usually involve comparisons of a non-epidural group, including many women who have comparatively quick, easy labours, with an epidural group many of whom are experiencing prolonged labour and may require planned instrumental delivery. Such selection bias makes any comparison invalid. Impact studies, comparing delivery outcome in a total parturient population before and after introduction of an epidural service, provide a much clearer picture of the effects of regional analgesia. Critics, however, point out the dangers of using historical controls as many changes in clinical practice, not just in pain relief, may affect the number of instrumental deliveries. Randomised prospective studies are the new gold standard of clinical research, but in labour such comparisons are difficult to perform as there is no effective alternative to offer the control group, recruits are reluctant and dropouts are frequent and unbalanced in the two groups. Moreover withholding epidural analgesia in a high-risk labour (see indications for regional analgesia in Chapter 8) may be regarded as unethical.

Caesarean section

There is a tendency amongst researchers to refer to the *risk* of caesarean section, or the *risk* of forceps delivery, as if these were natural occurrences like antepartum haemorrhage or pre-term labour. In any obstetric unit, the caesarean section rate depends above all on the habits of the local obstetricians, on their interpretation of fetal distress and failure to progress in labour and probably to a small degree on the characteristics and inclinations of the local childbearing population. Hence in the various studies purporting to examine the effects of epidural analgesia, caesarean section rates may vary between 10%[64] and 25%.[65] Instrumental delivery rates also vary widely, depending on local policies and attitudes towards the second stage. Since interventions, therefore, are determined by obstetricians rather than being *caused* by epidurals, objective outcome measures are needed to examine the true effects of central neural blockade. Indices that have been used include the strength and frequency of uterine contractions and the rate of cervical dilatation,[66] and the release of endogenous oxytocin in the second stage.[67] The use of such objective indices of the effects of neural blockade does not, however, obviate the need for randomisation with all its attendant problems. Moreover one may question the clinical relevance of such outcome measures. These shortcomings suggest that an *impact study* may not by comparison be such a blunt instrument. Among these, Bailey demonstrated no overall increase in the need for instrumental or caesarean delivery following the introduction of epidural analgesia in a

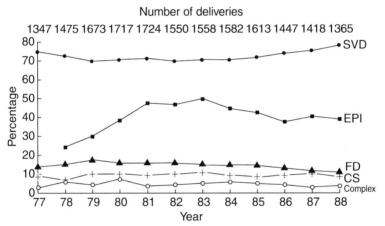

FIGURE 9.4—*The impact of an epidural analgesia service introduced in 1978 on the forceps and caesarean delivery rates. SVD, spontaneous vertex delivery; EPI, epidural; FD, forceps delivery; CS, caesarean section. (From Bailey[68] by permission of the author and publisher)*

single unit serving a stable community (Figure 9.4).[68] Other impact studies have similarly reported that an increase in the numbers receiving epidural analgesia was associated with no increase in the need for caesarean section (Table 9.3).[69–74]

Randomised studies comparing epidural with systemic analgesia have produced conflicting results. In an early study from Cardiff, Robinson and colleagues randomised women at 36 weeks' gestation to receive either epidural analgesia, using intermittent boluses of 0·5% bupivacaine, or intramuscular pethidine with inhalational analgesia.[75] Of the 386 mothers recruited antenatally, only 134 (36%) completed the study. The main reason for this was that those who deviated from the allocated analgesic

TABLE 9.3—*The impact of epidural analgesia on caesarean section rate*

| | Before | | After | |
	Epidural rate	CS (%)	Epidural rate	CS (%)
Bailey[68]	0	7.9	43	8.5
Robson et al[69]	10	4	45	5
Newman et al[70]	39.8	24.4	74.4	27.9
Gribble and Meier[71]	0	9	48	8
Larson[72]	0	28	32	23
Iglesias et al[73]	35	23	57	13
Gould[74]	2	10	42	12

technique were eliminated, instead of remaining to be grouped by intention to treat, a more modern approach. While some mothers randomised to receive epidural analgesia were admitted in advanced labour, too late to receive it, others who received pethidine had prolonged labour for which systemic analgesia was inadequate. Both situations biased the findings against epidurals, which were in the final analysis associated with longer labours and increased instrumental deliveries. Caesarean section was not mentioned in this study.

A smaller study from Denmark produced somewhat different findings.[76] Epidural top-ups of 0·375% bupivacaine were compared to intramuscular pethidine and inhalational analgesia in 112 mothers. Here 111 completed the study in which no significant differences in length of labour or mode of delivery were found. However, in this study epidural analgesia was discontinued in the second stage.

Thorp and colleagues, following retrospective surveys with predictable results,[77,78] attempted a prospective randomised trial comparing epidural infusions of 0·125% bupivacaine with intravenous pethidine and promethazine.[65] Although they originally planned to recruit 200 women, the trial was discontinued after 93 on the grounds that the findings made it unethical to continue. In the epidural group there was a significant prolongation of the first and second stages of labour, increased requirement for oxytocin and slower cervical dilatation. Caesarean section for dystocia but not fetal distress was significantly more common in the epidural group, as were instrumental vaginal deliveries. Further retrospective assessment of the results demonstrated that caesarean section was more likely if epidural analgesia was started before 5 cm cervical dilatation. This study was heavily criticised for the non-blinded selection of women for caesarean section, the use of oxytocin before randomisation, the absence of data on the time from randomisation until full dilatation and the strangely low section rate amongst those receiving pethidine (2·2%).

A recently published randomised trial compared bupivacaine/fentanyl epidural infusions and intravenous pethidine and promethazine.[79] Of the

1330 women randomised the dropout rate was 35%. Analysing on an intention to treat basis, the authors stated that the need for operative delivery (either caesarean section or forceps) for dystocia was 9% in the epidural group and 5% in those receiving pethidine. As in all these randomised studies, the quality of pain relief was significantly better in those who received epidural analgesia. The mechanism for the increased need for caesarean section for dystocia, if indeed the association exists, has yet to be described. Newton and colleagues compared myometrial activity in those receiving bupivacaine/fentanyl epidural infusions with a non-randomised group of controls receiving pethidine.[66] They reported no difference in myometrial contractility, although the need for oxytocin was greater and the rate of cervical dilatation slower in the epidural group. It has been suggested that preloading before regional analgesia with large volumes of intravenous fluid may inhibit the endogenous release of oxytocin.[80]

There is in some circles a reluctance to administer regional analgesia early in labour for fear of prolonging the first stage and increasing the caesarean section rate. Contractions in early labour may well be painful and to withhold effective analgesia is inhumane. Chestnut and colleagues investigated whether the timing of epidural analgesia influenced the need for caesarean section.[81,82] In studies of both spontaneous and induced labour women requesting epidural analgesia who were between 3 and 5 cm cervical dilatation were randomised to receive either plain bupivacaine or intravenous nalbuphine until they had reached 5 cm dilatation at which time epidural analgesia was provided for all. These prospective randomised studies showed that early epidural analgesia did not prolong labour nor did it increase the incidence of caesarean section or instrumental vaginal delivery, disproving the findings of Thorp and colleagues.[65]

Instrumental delivery

Although there is certainly an association between regional analgesia and instrumental delivery, their relationship is complex. Seven issues need to be addressed.

1 An appropriately run epidural service should catch the majority of mothers who are likely to need instrumental delivery. But does epidural analgesia *per se* add to their numbers?

The relationship between epidurals and instrumental deliveries has been the subject of numerous studies, but as with caesarean section (see above), the evidence is conflicting. Perhaps the main reason for this is the number of variables that may be relevant, such as the quality of analgesia, the use of oxytocin, and the timing and duration of active pushing (see below).

Retrospective studies suffer from selection bias and thus invariably show more instrumental deliveries in the epidural population. Randomised studies have demonstrated an increase in instrumental deliveries in those receiving epidurals,[65,75,79] but as with caesarean section, the decision to intervene is made by the obstetrician. Impact studies, again, provide far more useful information. In Bailey's study, despite the introduction of an epidural service used by over 70% of primiparous women, there was no significant increase in the number of instrumental deliveries (Figure 9.4).[68] There were similar findings at the National Maternity Hospital in Dublin, where the epidural rate increased from 10% in 1987 to 45% in 1992.[69] The spontaneous delivery rate was 82% in both years.

2 Removal of afferent stimuli blunts the reflex urge to bear down. Does discontinuing epidural analgesia in the second stage increase the spontaneous delivery rate?

A popular belief is that allowing analgesia to wear off during the second stage increases the number of spontaneous deliveries. Studies comparing epidural regimens have demonstrated that inferior second stage pain relief is associated with more spontaneous deliveries.[83] When Phillips and Thomas withheld second stage epidural top-ups of plain bupivacaine, however, they found mothers experienced significantly more pain but had fewer normal deliveries.[84] Chestnut and colleagues, in a series of double-blind studies, compared the effect of continuing an epidural infusion throughout the second stage with a saline placebo replacement at 8 cm dilatation. With 0·125% bupivacaine pain relief was better but the second stage prolonged and instrumental deliveries increased.[85] When the infusion was 0·0625% bupivacaine with fentanyl, however, continuation of analgesia did not prolong the second stage nor increase instrumental delivery, although analgesia was little better than in the saline controls.[86]

3 Motor block of the abdominal muscles may impair pushing, while relaxation of the pelvic floor may delay rotation of the vertex to occipito-anterior. Does reducing the local anaesthetic dosage to minimise motor block increase the spontaneous delivery rate?

Maintenance of epidural analgesia with bolus doses of 0·5% bupivacaine produces a dense block of sacral roots which may increase the incidence of malposition[87] and impair the mother's ability to push effectively.[83] It is now appreciated that labour analgesia can be achieved with far more dilute concentrations of local anaesthetic, thus avoiding dense motor block.

With the use of more dilute solutions only one study has linked motor block to increased instrumental delivery. Vertomenn and colleagues compared top-ups of 0·125% bupivacaine with or without 10 µg sufentanil.[88] The addition of sufentanil resulted in less motor block and fewer instrumental deliveries. However, in the second stage neither the quality of analgesia nor the obstetric management were reported. Other studies, in which the quality of sensory block has been standardised, have failed to find that decreasing motor blockade increases spontaneous delivery.[2,3,89-91]

4 In mothers receiving epidural analgesia, the normal second stage acceleration of uterine activity does not occur[92] as the increased endogenous oxytocin release provoked by afferent stimulation from the birth canal is inhibited.[67] Does administering exogenous oxytocin increase the spontaneous delivery rate?

Spontaneous delivery is unlikely if uterine activity is inadequate. In mothers receiving epidural analgesia it is imperative to assess the frequency, length, and strength of uterine contractions. Shennan and colleagues randomised primiparous mothers with epidural infusions of 0·125% bupivacaine at less than 6 cm cervical dilatation to receive oxytocin infusions or saline placebo.[93] Although length of the first stage was significantly shorter in the oxytocin group, there were no significant differences in the mode of delivery. Interestingly, over 50% of the control group received oxytocin augmentation after randomisation. Saunders and colleagues[94] randomised primiparous women having epidural bolus doses of 0·375% bupivacaine to receive oxytocin or placebo during the second stage and demonstrated a reduction in non-rotational forceps delivery in mothers receiving oxytocin. There were no significant differences between the groups in the incidence of rotational instrumental delivery.

5 With effective epidural analgesia, a well-hydrated mother and a normal fetal heart rate tracing, there is less need for haste in the second stage. Does delaying the start of active pushing increase the spontaneous delivery rate?

In women receiving regional analgesia the second stage is often diagnosed when the fetal head is high, in the transverse position and there is no desire to push. To start pushing at this time produces increasing metabolic disturbance[95] and maternal exhaustion usually occurs before spontaneous delivery is possible. It is therefore advisable to wait for descent of the fetal head and hopefully an urge to bear down.[96] Prolongation of the second stage is not harmful to the baby provided the mother is comfortable and well hydrated and there is no abnormality in fetal heart rate.[97] Not all studies, however, have found increased spontaneous delivery when pushing is delayed.[98]

6 In the presence of epidural analgesia, prolonged pushing is not associated with the same rate of deterioration of fetal acid base

status as with other methods of pain relief.[95] Does prolonging the active part of second stage increase the spontaneous delivery rate?

If there is no evidence of fetal distress and the mother is not fatigued, there should be no arbitrary limit to the duration of the active part of the second stage.[99] Once pushing starts, however, there must be ongoing descent of the fetal head. Intervention should only be necessary when there are signs of fetal or maternal distress or failure to progress. There is, however, little benefit to be gained from allowing the second stage to exceed a total of three hours.[100]

7 If instrumental delivery rate is increased, is this harmful to either mother or baby?

A well-conducted lift-out forceps or ventouse delivery should not produce adverse neonatal outcome.[101,102] More difficult rotational deliveries which may adversely affect the baby are thankfully becoming less common. The risk to the mother of instrumental delivery must be viewed against the effects of a prolonged second stage following which neurological, bladder and bowel problems have all been reported. As with the baby, the incidence of these sequelae is decreasing as the number of difficult and traumatic vaginal deliveries falls, although this is associated with an increased number of caesarean sections.

Effects of regional blockade on the baby

Mothers are naturally anxious about possible adverse effects on the baby of any procedures performed during childbirth. Regional analgesia and anaesthesia may in theory affect the baby either directly by the placental transfer of maternally administered drugs or indirectly by changes in placental perfusion, maternal acid–base status or the progress of labour. When examining these effects two questions need to be answered. Does regional analgesia have significant effects on the baby and do differences in regional techniques confer a greater or lesser risk to the baby?

Pharmacological effects

The lipophilic drugs used to provide regional analgesia cross the placenta readily. However, adverse effects on the baby will only be seen if maternal systemic levels reach the toxic threshold. If lignocaine is used to provide continuous epidural analgesia, toxic effects may be observed in both mother and baby[103] and its use for continuous epidural analgesia in labour is not recommended. Bupivacaine has a longer duration of action, so systemic toxicity is unlikely and indeed no difference in neonatal outcome is observed whether it is given epidurally or spinally.[104] The effects of ropivacaine are still under evaluation.

Opioids have more potential to produce neonatal depression, but if given in appropriate dose by infusion, adverse effects are unlikely.[2,105] If, however, large or repeated doses are given, neonatal depression may arise.[106,107]

Indirect effects

Local anaesthetics block preganglionic sympathetic fibres producing vasodilatation. If vasodilatation is widespread, hypotension may result which may impair placental gas exchange and result in fetal acidosis. Providing that hypotension is avoided, by adequate preloading and positioning, regional anaesthesia improves intervillous blood flow.[13] Painful labour increases maternal catecholamine levels, causing vasoconstriction in uterine vessels. Maternal hyperventilation and hypocarbia further constrict uterine vasculature and impair gas exchange (see Figure 1.2). Effective pain relief using regional techniques reduces catecholamine levels and hyperventilation, thus improving placental blood flow.[12]

Assessment of the baby during labour

There are various ways in which the effects of regional analgesia on the baby, both in utero and neonatally, may be judged, although none provides a completely reliable assessment.

Fetal heart rate   Continuous fetal heart rate monitoring is widely used in labour, although its success in reducing fetal mortality and morbidity has yet to be clearly demonstrated.[108] Despite this, cardiotocographic (CTG) monitoring is still recommended for all mothers receiving regional analgesia.[109] Changes in fetal heart rate patterns, both improvement and deterioration, have been observed in the 30 minutes after the loading dose.[110] Abboud and colleagues reported occasional decelerations in the fetuses of mothers receiving bupivacaine, chloroprocaine or lignocaine, most frequently in the former.[111] Others have found no significant differences in fetal heart traces between bupivacaine, lignocaine or ropivacaine.[112,113] Nor have any differences been observed when plain local anaesthetic solutions have been compared to those of low dose combined with opioids.[2,114] Providing CTG changes do not reflect poor placental perfusion resulting from maternal hypotension, their relevance to fetal outcome is probably random and unimportant.[115]

Intervillous blood flow   The effect of epidural analgesia on uteroplacental blood flow was originally assessed by radionuclide methods. Placental clearance of radioactive xenon was measured following inhalation or intravenous injection. Using this technique epidural analgesia produced a significant increase in intervillous blood flow in the absence of hypotension[116] and did not significantly reduce intervillous blood flow even in the presence of maternal hypotension.[117] Moreover, blood flow was more consistently increased in those with pre-eclampsia.[118]

With concerns over the use of radioactive compounds in the pregnant population, Doppler ultrasound superseded radionuclide methods of

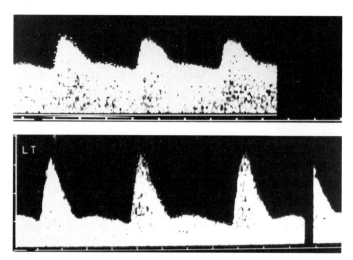

FIGURE 9.5—*Doppler flow/velocity waveforms from the uterine artery in the third trimester:* upper, *normal pattern with good flow during diastole;* lower, *abnormal, greater difference between systolic and diastolic flow*

assessing uteroplacental blood flow (Figure 9.5). Blood velocity waveforms can be recorded non-invasively from uterine, umbilical, and major fetal vessels. From these waveforms, indices of resistance can be derived, and if vessel cross-section is measured, flow can be estimated.

It would appear that regional analgesia lowers resistance to uterine blood flow and has a neutral effect on fetal blood flow provided hypotension is avoided.[119–121] The use of adrenaline in local anaesthetic solutions appears to have little effect on intervillous blood flow in normal labour.[116,122] However, in pre-eclamptic mothers it is probably best avoided, as the sensitivity to catecholamines is increased.

When hypotension occurs, the vasopressor of choice is ephedrine. It is an indirectly acting sympathomimetic with both α and β effects causing negligible increase in uterine vascular resistance and no apparent detrimental effect on the baby.[123] By contrast, the pure α agonist phenylephrine has been demonstrated to increase uterine artery resistance.[124,125]

Fetal blood sampling Sampling of fetal blood during labour provides a more accurate assessment of fetal well-being than does the CTG. The deterioration in fetal blood gases seen in the first stage of labour with systemic analgesia does not occur when epidural blockade with bupivacaine is used.[126] Deterioration is also delayed by epidural bupivacaine in the second stage, especially in the absence of active pushing.[95,127] Epidural analgesia may improve fetal haemoglobin saturation by reducing maternal hyperventilation,[128] so reducing the affinity of maternal haemoglobin for oxygen (Bohr effect) and enhancing oxygen supply to the fetus.

Others Other minimally invasive techniques are being developed to assess fetal welfare. Continuous fetal oximetry, fetal pH and transcutaneous oxygen and carbon dioxide measurement are all currently under evaluation, but as yet their role in obstetric practice remains uncertain.

Assessment of the baby after delivery

Apgar scores Apgar scoring has been used widely to assess the condition of the newborn. The score does, however, lack sufficient sensitivity to pick up subtle changes that may result from sensible maternal drug administration during labour. No significant differences in Apgar scores have been demonstrated in randomised trials where epidural analgesia, with either bupivacaine[65,76] or bupivacaine with opioid,[79] has been compared to systemic analgesia. However, in certain high-risk situations, such as twins[129] and low birthweight infants,[130] epidurals have been associated with increased Apgar scores compared to systemic analgesia. When used to assess babies after caesarean section, higher Apgar scores have been demonstrated with regional than with general anaesthesia.[131-133]

Umbilical cord blood analysis Umbilical artery and vein blood gas and acid–base values provide a retrospective estimate of peripartum asphyxia. Studies of umbilical cord blood have again shown no detrimental effects of regional analgesia, using bupivacaine either alone or supplemented.[65,79,128]

Neurobehavioural scores Neurobehavioural status of the newborn has been developed in an attempt to evaluate the effects of maternal drug administration on the baby. The Brazelton Neonatal Behavioural Assessment Scale (BNBAS)[134] and the Scanlon Early Neonatal Neurobehavioural Scale (ENNS)[135] are both somewhat complex and time-consuming and so the more easily performed Neurologic and Adaptive Capacity Score (NACS) is now most commonly used (Figure 9.6).[136] The score is based on passive and active tone, primitive reflexes, and general behaviour and is designed to distinguish between the depressant effects of drugs and perinatal asphyxia or birth trauma.

171

	Score	0	1	2
1 Scarf sign		encircles the neck	elbow slightly passes midline	elbow does not reach midline
2 Recoil of elbows		absent	slow; weak	brisk; reproducible
3 Popliteal angle		>110°	100–110°	≤90°
4 Recoil of lower limbs		absent	slow; weak	brisk; reproducible
5 Active contraction of neck flexors (from lying position)		absent or abnormal	difficult	good; head is maintained in the axis of the body
6 Active contraction of neck extensors (from leaning forward position)		absent or abnormal	difficult	good; head is maintained in the axis of the body
7 Palmar grasp		absent	weak	excellent; reproducible
8 Response to traction (following palmar grasp)		absent	lifts part of the body weight	lifts all the body weight
9 Supporting reaction (upright position)		absent	incomplete; transitory	strong; supports all body weight
10 Automatic walking		absent	difficult to obtain	perfect; reproducible
11 Sucking		absent	weak	perfect; synchronous with swallowing
12 Moro reflex		absent	weak; incomplete	perfect; complete
13 Alertness		coma	lethargy or hyperexcitability	normal
14 Crying		absent	abnormal (poor or excessive)	normal
15 Motor activity		absent	diminished or excessive	normal
Neurological sub-total				
16 Response to sound		absent	mild	vigorous
17 Habituation to sound		absent	7–12 stimuli	≤6 stimuli
18 Response to light		absent	mild	brisk blink or startle
19 Habituation to light		absent	7–12 stimuli	≤6 stimuli
20 Consolability		absent	difficult	easy
Adaptive capacity sub-total				

Total score [ ] **at** **minutes of life**

FIGURE 9.6—*The Neurological and Adaptive Capacity Score (NACS) in full-term newborns. (From Amiel Tison et al.[136] with permission)*

172

Neurologic and Adaptive Capacity Scoring has not revealed any detrimental effects of regional anaesthesia, either with bupivacaine alone or in low dose combination with opioid. Indeed Kangas Saarela and colleagues demonstrated better scores amongst neonates whose mothers had received epidural analgesia than amongst unmedicated controls.[137] Neonatal depression has been observed with excessively large doses of epidural alfentanil ($30\,\mu g/kg + 30\,\mu g\,kg^{-1}h^{-1}$)[106] and sufentanil ($80\,\mu g$).[107] Epidural opioids might be expected, first and foremost, to depress neonatal respiration as they do when given systemically to the mother. Neurobehavioural studies, however, may not be appropriate to detect minor degrees of respiratory depression. More recent studies of transcutaneous oxygen and carbon dioxide tension in the newborn have revealed no significant or clinically important differences among babies born to mothers receiving plain bupivacaine and those who received low dose bupivacaine with fentanyl by infusion.[105]

References

1 Murphy JD, Henderson K, Bowden MI, Lewis M, Cooper GM. Bupivacaine versus bupivacaine plus fentanyl for epidural analgesia: effect on maternal satisfaction. *BMJ* 1991;**301**:564–7.

2 Russell R, Reynolds F. Epidural infusion of low-dose bupivacaine and opioid in labour. Does reducing motor block increase the spontaneous delivery rate? *Anaesthesia* 1996; **51**:266–73.

3 Collis RE, Davies DWL, Aveling W. Randomised comparison of combined spinal-epidural with standard epidural analgesia in labour. *Lancet* 1995;**345**:1413–16.

4 Morgan BM, Bulpitt CJ, Clifton P, Lewis PJ. Analgesia and satisfaction in childbirth (The Queen Charlotte's 1000 Mother Survey). *Lancet* 1982;**ii**:808–10.

5 Buggy D, Hughes N, Gardiner J. Posterior column sensory impairment during ambulatory extradural analgesia in labour. *Br J Anaesth* 1994;**73**:540–2.

6 Parry MG, Bawa GPS, Poulton B, Fernando R. Dorsal column function in parturients receiving epidural and combined spinal epidural for labour and elective caesarean section. *Int J Obstet Anesth* 1996;**5**:213.

7 Camann WR, Horvet LA, Hughes N, Bader AM, Datta S. Maternal temperature regulation during extradural analgesia for labour. *Br J Anaesth* 1991;**67**:565–8.

8 Fusi L, Maresh MJA, Steer PJ, Beard RW. Maternal pyrexia associated with the use of epidural analgesia in labour. *Lancet* 1989;**i**:1250–2.

9 Moore J. The effects of analgesia and anaesthesia on maternal stress response. In: Reynolds F, ed. *Effects on the baby of maternal analgesia and anaesthesia*. London: Baillière Tindall, 1993:148–62.

10 Morishima HO, Pederson H, Finster M. The influence of maternal psychological stress on the fetus. *Am J Obstet Gynecol* 1978;**131**:286–90.

11 Westgren M, Lindahl SGE, Norden NE. Maternal and fetal endocrine stress response at vaginal delivery with and without epidural block. *J Perinat Med* 1986;**14**:235–41.

12 Shnider SM, Abboud TK, Artal R. Maternal catecholamines decrease during labor after epidural anesthesia. *Am J Obstet Gynecol* 1983;**147**:13–15.

13 Hollmen AI, Jouppila R, Jouppila P, Koivula A, Vierola H. Effects of extradural analgesia using bupivacaine or 2-chloroprocaine on intervillous blood flow during normal labour. *Br J Anaesth* 1982;**54**:837–42.

14 Jouppila R, Jouppila P, Hollmen A, Koivula A. Epidural analgesia and placental blood flow during labour in pregnancies complicated by hypertension. *Br J Obstet Gynaecol* 1979;**86**:969–72.

15 Abboud T, Artal A, Sarkis F, Henriksen EH, Kammula RK. Sympathoadrenal activity: maternal, fetal and neonatal responses after epidural anesthesia in the pre-eclamptic parturient. *Am J Obstet Gynecol* 1982;**144:**915–18.

16 Dray A. Epidural opiates and urinary retention: new models provide new insights (Editorial). *Anesthesiology* 1988;**68:**323–4.

17 Durrant PAC, Yaksh TL. Drug effects on urinary bladder tone during spinal morphine induced inhibition of micturition reflex in unanesthetised rats. *Anesthesiology* 1988;**68:** 325–34.

18 Russell R, Reynolds F. Long term effects of epidural analgesia. In: Bogod D, ed. Obstetric anaesthesia *Clin Anaesthesiol* 1995;**9:**607–22.

19 Grove LH. Backache, headache and bladder dysfunction after delivery. *Br J Anaesth* 1973;**45:**1147–9.

20 Tessler MJ, Weisel S, Wahba RM, Quance DR. A comparison of simple identification tests to distinguish cerebrospinal fluid from local anaesthetic solution. *Anaesthesia* 1994; **49:**821–2.

21 Crawford JS. Some maternal complications of epidural analgesia for labour. *Anaesthesia* 1985;**40:**1219–25.

22 Gupta A, Enlund G, Bengtsson M, Sjoberg F. Spinal anaesthesia for caesarean section following epidural analgesia in labour: a relative contraindication. *Int J Obstet Anesth* 1994;**3:**153–6.

23 Glosten B. Obstetric anesthesia risk: a review of recent literature. *Int J Obstet Anesth* 1994;**3:**7–12.

24 Halpern S, Preston R. Postdural puncture headache and spinal needle design: meta-analysis. *Anesthesiology* 1994;**81:**1376–83.

25 Meikeljohn BH. The effect of rotating the epidural needle. *Anaesthesia* 1987;**42:**1180–2.

26 Stride PC, Cooper GM. Dural taps revisited. *Anaesthesia* 1993;**48:**247–55.

27 Thorburn J, Moir DD. Bupivacaine toxicity in association with extradural anaesthesia for caesarean section. *Br J Anaesth* 1984;**56:**551–2.

28 Crawford JS, Davies P, Lewis M. Some aspects of epidural block provided for caesarean section. *Anaesthesia* 1986;**41:**1039–46.

29 Laishley RS Morgan BM, Reynolds F. Effect of adrenaline on extradural anaesthesia and plasma bupivacaine concentrations during caesarean section. *Br J Anaesth* 1988;**60:** 180–6.

30 Ong BY, Cohen MM, Esmail A, Cumming M, Kozody R, Palahniuk RJ. Paresthesias and motor dysfunction after labor and delivery. *Anesth Analg* 1987;**66:**18–22.

31 Donaldson JO. *Neurology of pregnancy*, 2nd edn. Philadelphia: Saunders, 1989.

32 Holdcroft A, Gibberd FB, Hargrove RL, Dawkins DF, Dellaports CI. Neurological complications associated with pregnancy. *Br J Anaesth* 1995;**75:**522–6.

33 Scott DB, Hibbard BM. Serious non-fatal complications associated with extradural block in obstetric practice. *Br J Anaesth* 1990:**64:**537–41.

34 Scott DB, Tunstall ME. Serious complications associated with epidural/spinal blockade in obstetrics. *Int J Obstet Anesth* 1995:**4:**133–9.

35 Rendell-Baker L. Paraplegia from accidental injection of potassium chloride solution. *Anaesthesia* 1985;**40:**912–13.

36 Sgchirlanzoni A, Marazzi R, Pareyson D, Oliveri A, Bracchi M. Epidural anaesthesia and spinal arachnoiditis. *Anaesthesia* 1989;**44:**317–21.

37 Reynolds F. Maternal sequelae of childbirth. *Br J Anaesth* 1995;**75:**515–17.

38 Ferguson FR, Watkins KH. Paralysis of the bladder and associated neurological sequelae of spinal anaesthesia (cauda equina syndrome). *Br J Surg* 1937;**25:**735–42.

39 Kennedy F, Effron A, Perry G. The grave spinal cord paralyses caused by spinal anesthesia. *Surg Gynecol Obstet* 1950;**91:**385–98.

40 Hutter CDD. The Wolley and Roe case: a reassessment. *Anaesthesia* 1990;**45:**859–64.

41 Rigler ML, Drasner K, Krejcie TC *et al.* Cauda equina syndrome after continuous spinal anaesthesia. *Anesth Analg* 1991;**72:**275–81.

42 Snyder R, Hui G, Flugstad P, Viarengo C. More cases of possible neurotoxicity associated with single subarachnoid injections of 5% hyperbaric lidocaine. *Anesth Analg* 1994;**78:** 411.

43 Fenerty J, Sonner J, Sakura S, Drasner K. Transient radicular pain following spinal anesthesia: review of the literature and report of a case involving 2% lignocaine. *Int J Obstet Anesth* 1996;**5**:32–5.

44 Reisner LS, Hochman BN, Plumer MH. Persistant neurologic deficit and adhesive arachnoiditis following intrathecal 2-chloroprocaine injection. *Anesth Analg* 1980;**59**: 452–4.

45 Drasner K, Rigler ML, Sessler DI, Stoller ML. Cauda equina syndrome following intended epidural anesthesia. *Anesth Analg* 1992;**77**:582–5.

46 Cheng A. Intended epidural anesthesia as possible cause of cauda equina syndrome. *Anesth Analg* 1993;**78**:157–9.

47 Craig DB, Habin GG. Flaccid paralysis following obstetrical anesthesia: the possible role of benzyl alcohol. *Anesth Analg* 1977;**56**:219–21.

48 Braham J, Saia A. Neurological complications of epidural analgesia. *BMJ* 1958;**ii**:657.

49 Harding SA, Collis RE, Morgan BM. Meningitis after combined spinal-extradural anaesthesia in obstetrics. *Br J Anaesth* 1994;**73**:545–7.

50 Ackerman WE, Juneja MM, Knapp RK. Maternal paraparesis after epidural anesthesia and cesarean section. *South Med J* 1990;**83**:695–7.

51 Eastwood DW. Anterior spinal artery syndrome after epidural anesthesia in a pregnant diabetic patient with scleroderma. *Anesth Analg* 1991;**73**:90–1.

52 Yoshii WY, Rottman RL, Rosenblatt RM *et al.* Epidural catheter induced traumatic radiculopathy in obstetrics: one center's experience. *Regional Anesth* 1994;**19**:132–5.

53 Silva M, Mallinson C, Reynolds F. Sciatic nerve palsy following childbirth. *Anaesthesia* 1996;**51**:1144–8.

54 Crawford JS. Lumbar epidural block in labour: a clinical analysis. *Br J Anaesth* 1972; **44**:66–74.

55 Shutt LE, Valentine SJ, Wee MYK, Page RJ, Prosser A, Thomas TA. Spinal anaesthesia for caesarean section: comparison of 22-gauge and 25-gauge Whitacre needles with 26-gauge Quincke needles. *Br J Anaesth* 1992;**69**:589–94.

56 MacArthur C, Lewis M, Knox EG, Crawford JS. Epidural anaesthesia and long term backache after childbirth. *BMJ* 1990;**301**:9–12.

57 Russell R, Groves P, Taub N, O'Dowd J, Reynolds F. Assessing long-term backache after childbirth. *BMJ* 1993;**306**:1299–302.

58 Russell R, Dundas R, Reynolds F. Long-term backache after childbirth: prospective search for causative factors. *BMJ* 1996;**312**:1384–8.

59 Macarthur A, Macarthur C, Weeks S. Epidural anesthesia and long-term back pain after delivery: a prospective cohort study. *BMJ* 1995;**311**:1336–9.

60 Breen TW, Ransil BJ, Groves PA, Oriol NE. Factors associated with back pain after childbirth. *Anesthesiology* 1994;**81**:29–34.

61 Nimmo WS, Wilson J, Prescott LF. Narcotic analgesia and delayed gastric emptying during labour. *Lancet* 1975;**i**:890–3.

62 Wright PMC, Allen RW Moore J, Donelly JP. Gastric emptying during lumbar extradural analgesia in labour; effect of fentanyl supplementation. *Br J Anaesth* 1992;**68**:248–51.

63 Porter J, Bonello E, Reynolds F. The influence of epidural fentanyl infusion on gastric emptying in labour. *Int J Obstet Anesth* 1995;**4**:261.

64 Naulty JS, March MG, Leavitt KL, Smith R, Urso PR. Effects of changes in labor analgesia on practice outcome. *Anesthesiology* 1992;**77**:A979.

65 Thorp JA, Hu DH, Albin RM, *et al.* The effect of intrapartum epidural analgesia on nulliparous labor: a randomized, controlled, prospective study. *Am J Obstet Gynecol* 1993;**169**:851–8.

66 Newton ER, Schroeder BC, Knape KG, Bennett BL. Epidural analgesia and uterine function. *Obstet Gynecol* 1995;**85**:749–55.

67 Goodfellow CF, Hull MGR, Swaab DF, Dogterom J, Buijs RM. Oxytocin deficiency at delivery with epidural analgesia. *Br J Obstet Gynaecol* 1983;**90**:214–9.

68 Bailey PW. Epidural analgesia and the management of the second stage of labour: a failure to progress. In: Reynolds F, ed. *Epidural and spinal blockade in obstetrics*. London: Baillière Tindall, 1990:59–72.

69 Robson M, Boylan P, McParland P, McQuillan C, O'Neill MO. Epidural analgesia need not influence the spontaneous delivery rate. *Am J Obstet Gynecol* 1993;**168**:364.

70 Newman LM, Perez EC, Krolick TJ, Ivankovich AD. Labor analgesia, cesarean anesthesia and cesarean delivery rates for 18 000 deliveries from 1988 through 1994. *Anesthesiology* 1995;**83**:A968.

71 Gribble RK, Meier PR. Effects of epidural analgesia on the primary cesarean rate. *Obstet Gynecol* 1991;**78**:231-4.

72 Larson DD. The effect of initiating an obstetric anesthesiology service on rate of cesarean section and rate of forceps delivery. Society for Obstetric Anesthesia and Perinatology Annual Meeting, Charleston, SC, 1992:13.

73 Iglesias S, Burn R, Saunders LD. Reducing the cesarean section rate in a rural community hospital. *Can Med Assoc J* 1991;**145**:1459-64.

74 Gould DB. Are today's epidurals the 12% solution. *Anesthesiology* 1995;**82**:311-12.

75 Robinson JO, Rosen M, Evans JM, Revill SI, David H, Rees GAD. Maternal opinion about analgesia in labour: a controlled trial between epidural block and intramuscular pethidine combined with inhalation. *Anaesthesia* 1980;**35**:1173-81.

76 Philipsen T, Jensen NH. Epidural block or parenteral pethidine as analgesic in labour; a randomized study concerning progress in labour and instrumental deliveries. *Eur J Obstet Gynaecol Reprod Biol* 1989;**30**:27-33.

77 Thorp JA, Parisi VM, Boylan PC, Johnston DA. The effect of continuous epidural analgesia on cesarean section for dystocia in nulliparous women. *Am J Obstet Gynecol* 1989;**161**:670-5.

78 Thorp JA, Eckert LO, Ang MS, Johnston DA, Peaceman AM, Parisi VM. Epidural analgesia and cesarean section for dystocia; risk factors for nulliparous. *Am J Perinatol* 1991;**8**:402-10.

79 Ramin SM, Gambling DR, Lucas MJ, Sharma SK, Sidawi JE, Leveno KJ. Randomized trial of epidural versus intravenous analgesia during labor. *Obstet Gynecol* 1995;**86**:783-9.

80 Cheek TG, Samuels P, Miller F, Tobin M, Gutsche BB. Normal saline i.v. fluid load decreases uterine activity in active labour. *Br J Anaesth* 1996;**77**:632-5.

81 Chestnut DH, Vincent RD, McGrath JM, Choi WW, Bates JN. Does early administration of epidural analgesia affect obstetric outcome in nulliparous women who are receiving intravenous oxytocin? *Anesthesiology* 1994;**80**:1193-200.

82 Chestnut DH, McGrath JM, Vincent RD *et al*. Does early administration of epidural analgesia affect obstetric outcome in nulliparous women who are in spontaneous labor? *Anesthesiology* 1994;**80**:1201-8.

83 Thorburn J, Moir DD. Extradural analgesia: the influence of volume and concentration of bupivacaine on the mode of delivery, analgesia efficacy and motor blockade. *Br J Anaesth* 1981;**53**:933-9.

84 Phillips KC, Thomas TA. Second stage of labour with or without extradural analgesia. *Anaesthesia* 1983;**38**:972-6.

85 Chestnut DH, Vanderwalker GE, Owen CL, Bates JN, Choi WW. The influence of continuous epidural bupivacaine analgesia on the second stage of labor and method of delivery in nulliparous women. *Anesthesiology* 1987;**66**:774-80.

86 Chestnut DH, Laszewski LJ, Pollack KL, Bates JN, Mango NK, Choi WW. Continuous epidural infusion of 0·0625% bupivacaine-0·0002% fentanyl during the second stage of labor. *Anesthesiology* 1990;**72**:613-19.

87 Hoult IJ, MacLennan AH, Carrie LES. Lumbar epidural analgesia in labour: relation to fetal malposition and instrumental delivery. *BMJ* 1977;**i**:14-16.

88 Vertommen JD, Vandermeulen E, Van Aken H, *et al*. The effects of the addition of sufentanil to 0·125% bupivacaine on the quality of analgesia during labor and on the incidence of instrumental deliveries. *Anesthesiology* 1991;**74**:809-14.

89 Bailey CR, Ruggier R, Findley IL. Diamorphine-bupivacaine mixture compared with plain bupivacaine for analgesia. *Br J Anaesth* 1994;**72**:58-61.

90 Phillips GH. Continuous infusion epidural analgesia in labor. *Anesth Analg* 1988;**67**:462-5.

91 Rodriguez J, Abboud TK, Reyes A *et al*. Continuous infusion epidural anesthesia during labor: a randomised double-blind comparison of 0·0625% bupivacaine/0·002% butorphanol and 0·125% bupivacaine. *Regional Anesth* 1990;**15**:300-3.

92 Bates RC, Helm CW, Duncan A, Edmonds DK. Uterine activity in the second stage of labour and the effect of epidural analgesia. *Br J Obstet Gynaecol* 1985;**92**:1246–50.

93 Shennan AH, Smith R, Browne D, Edmonds DK, Morgan B. The elective use of oxytocin infusion during labour in nulliparous women using epidural analgesia. *Int J Obstet Anesth* 1995;**4**:78–81.

94 Saunders NJStG, Spiby H, Gilbert L *et al.* Oxytocin infusion during the second stage of labour in primiparous women using epidural analgesia: a randomised double blind placebo controlled trial. *BMJ* 1989;**299**:1423–6.

95 Pearson JF, Davies P. The effect of continuous lumbar epidural analgesia upon fetal acid-base status during the second stage of labour. *J Obstet Gynaecol Br Commonw* 1974; **81**:975–9.

96 Maresh M, Choong KH, Beard RW. Delayed pushing with lumbar epidural analgesia in labour. *Br J Obstet Gynaecol* 1983;**90**:623–7.

97 Cohen WR. Influence of the duration of the second stage on perinatal outcome and puerperal morbidity. *Obstet Gynecol* 1977;**48**:266–9.

98 Buxton EJ, Redman CWE, Obhrai M. Delayed pushing with lumbar epidural in labour – does it increase the incidence of spontaneous delivery? *J Obstet Gynaecol* 1988;**8**: 258–61.

99 Crawford JS. *Principles and practice of obstetric anaesthesia.* Oxford: Blackwell Scientific Publications, 1984.

100 Kadar N, Cruddas M, Campbell S. Estimating the probability of spontaneous delivery conditional on time spent in the second stage. *Br J Obstet Gynaecol* 1986;**93**:568–76.

101 McBride WG, Black BP, Brown CJ, Dolby RM, Murray AD, Thomas DB. Method of delivery and developmental outcome at five years of age. *Med J Aust* 1979;**1**:301–4.

102 Friedman EA, Sachtleben-Murray MR, Dahrouge D, Neff RK. Long-term effects of labor and delivery on offspring: a matched-pair analysis. *Am J Obstet Gynecol* 1984;**150**: 941–5.

103 Reynolds F, Taylor G. Maternal and neonatal concentrations of bupivacaine: a comparison with lignocaine during continuous extradural analgesia. *Anaesthesia* 1970;**25**:14–23.

104 Jani K, McEvedy B, Harris S, Samaan A. Maternal and neonatal bupivacaine concentrations after spinal and extradural anaesthesia for caesarean section. *Br J Anaesth* 1989;**62**:226–7.

105 Porter J, Reynolds F. The effect of epidural opioids on neonatal respiration. *Int J Obstet Anesth* 1996;**5**:210.

106 Heytens L, Cammu H, Cammu F. Extradural analgesia during labour using alfentanil. *Br J Anaesth* 1987;**59**:331–7.

107 Capogna G, Celleno D, Tomasetti M. Maternal analgesia and neonatal neurobehavioral effects of epidural sufentanil for cesarean section. *Abstracts of the Congress of Regional Anesthesia* 1989;**14**:24.

108 Groves PA, Oriol NE. How useful is intrapartum electronic fetal heart rate monitoring? *Int J Obstet Anesth* 1995;**4**:161–7.

109 Obstetric Anaesthetists' Association Working Party. Recommended minimum standards for obstetric anaesthesia services. *Int J Obstet Anesth* 1995;**4**:125–8.

110 Rickford WJK, Reynolds F. Epidural analgesia in labour and maternal posture. *Anaesthesia* 1983;**38**:1169–74.

111 Abboud TK, Afrasiabi A, Sarkis F *et al.* Continuous infusion epidural analgesia in parturients receiving bupivacaine, chloroprocaine or lidocaine–maternal, fetal and neonatal effects. *Anesth Analg* 1984;**63**:421–8.

112 Milaszkiewicz R, Payne N, Loughnan B, Blackett A, Barber N, Carli F. Continuous extradural infusion of lignocaine 0·75% vs bupivacaine 0·125% in primiparae: quality of analgesia and influence on labour. *Anaesthesia* 1992;**47**:1042–6.

113 McCrae AF, Jowiak H, McClure JH. Comparison of ropivacaine and bupivacaine in extradural analgesia for the relief of pain in labour. *Br J Anaesth* 1995;**74**:261–265.

114 Cohen SE, Tan S, Albright GA, Halpern J. Epidural fentanyl/bupivacaine mixtures for obstetric analgesia. *Anesthesiology* 1987;**67**:403–7.

115 Reynolds F. Effects on the baby of conduction blockade in obstetrics. In: Reynolds F, ed. *Epidural and spinal blockade in obstetrics.* London, Baillière Tindall, 1990:205–218.

116 Jouppila R, Jouppila P, Kuikka J. Placental blood flow during caesarean section under lumbar extradural analgesia. *Br J Anaesth* 1978;**50**:275–9.

117 Huovinen K, Lehtovirta P, Forss M, Kivalo I, Teramo K. Changes in placental intervillous blood flow measured by the [133]xenon method during lumbar epidural block for elective caesarean section. *Acta Anaesth Scand* 1979;**23**:529–33.

118 Jouppila P, Jouppila R, Hollmen A, Koivula A. Lumbar epidural analgesia to improve intervillous blood flow during labor in severe preeclampsia. *Obstet Gynecol* 1982;**59**:158–61.

119 Hollmen A. Effect of regional anaesthesia on placental blood flow. In: Reynolds F, ed. *Effects on the baby of maternal anaesthesia and analgesia*. London: Saunders, 1993:67–87.

120 Marx GF, Shashikant P, Berman JA, Farmakides G, Schulman H. Umbilical blood flow velocity waveform in different maternal positions and with epidural analgesia. *Obstet Gynecol* 1986;**68**:61–4.

121 Lindblad A, Marsal K, Vernersson E, Renck H. Fetal circulation during epidural analgesia for caesarean section. *BMJ* 1984;**288**:1329–30.

122 Alahuhta S, Rasanen J, Jouppila R, Jouppila P, Hollmen A. Effects of extradural bupivacaine with adrenaline for caesarean section on uteroplacental and fetal circulation. *Br J Anaesth* 1991;**67**:678–82.

123 Hollmen AI, Jouppila R, Albright GA. Intervillous blood flow during caesarean section with prophylactic ephedrine and epidural analgesia. *Acta Anaesth Scand* 1984;**28**:396–400.

124 Rasanen J, Alahuhta S, Kangas-Saarela T, Jouppila R, Jouppila P. The effects of ephedrine and etilefrine on uterine and fetal blood flow and on fetal myocardial function during spinal anaesthesia for caesarean section. *Int J Obstet Anesth* 1991;**1**:3–8.

125 Alahuhta S, Rasanen J, Jouppila P, Jouppila R, Hollmen AI. Ephedrine and phenylephrine for avoiding maternal hypotension due to spinal anaesthesia for caesarean section. *Int J Obstet Anesth* 1992;**1**:129–34.

126 Pearson JF, Davies P. The effect of continuous lumbar epidural analgesia upon fetal acid-base status during the first stage of labour. *J Obstet Gynaecol Br Commonwlth* 1974;**81**:971–4.

127 Thalme B, Belfrage P, Raabe N. Lumbar epidural analgesia in labour: I. Acid-base balance and clinical condition of the mother, fetus and newborn child. *Acta Obstet Gynecol Scand* 1974;**53**:27–35.

128 Deckardt R, Fernbacher PM, Schneider KTM, Graeff H. Maternal arterial oxygen saturation during labor and delivery: pain dependent alterations and effects on the newborn. *Obstet Gynecol* 1987;**70**:21–5.

129 Crawford JS. A prospective study of 200 consecutive twin deliveries. *Anaesthesia* 1987;**42**:33–43.

130 Osbourne GK, Patel NB, Howat RCL. A comparison of outcome of low birthweight pregnancy in Glasgow and Dundee. *Health Bull (Edinb)* 1984;**42**:68–77.

131 Ong BY, Cohen MM, Palahniuk RJ. Anesthesia for cesarean section – effects on neonates. *Anesth Analg* 1989;**68**:270–5.

132 Marx GF, Luykx WM, Cohen S. Fetal-neonatal status following caesarean section for fetal distress. *Br J Anaesth* 1984;**56**:1009–13.

133 Evans CM, Murphy JF, Gray OP, Rosen M. Epidural versus general anaesthesia for elective caesarean section. Effect on Apgar score and acid-base status of the newborn. *Anaesthesia* 1989;**44**:778–82.

134 Brazelton TB. *Neonatal Behavioral Assessment Scale*, 2nd edn. (Clinics in Developmental Medicine, No. 88). London: Blackwell, 1984:125.

135 Scanlon JW, Brown WU, Weiss JB, Alper MH. Neurobehavioral responses of newborn infants after maternal epidural anesthesia. *Anesthesiology* 1974;**40**:121–8.

136 Amiel Tison C, Barrier G, Shnider SM, Levinson G, Hughes SC, Stefani SJ. A new neurologic and adaptive capacity scoring system for evaluating obstetric medications in full term newborns. *Anesthesiology* 1982;**56**:340–50.

137 Kangas Saarela T, Jouppila R, Jouppila P et al. The effect of segmental epidural analgesia on neurobehavioural responses of newborn infants. *Acta Anaesth Scand* 1987;**31**:347–51.

10: Practical procedures

Consent

Increasing consumer demand for information and choice during childbirth and the rising tide of litigation against medical staff has made the issue of consent one of great importance. The key questions are: what, when and how should women be told about the risks and benefits of both regional and general anaesthesia?[1]

Informed consent must allow the patient to understand the nature, consequences and complications of the procedure to be performed. Which of various complications it is necessary to mention to women is an area of debate. For epidural analgesia in labour, most anaesthetists both in the UK and USA would discuss quality of pain relief, benefit to the baby, advantages for operative delivery and the risk of headache after accidental dural puncture.[2] Discussion of other genuine complications such as accidental intravenous or intrathecal injection is rarely considered whereas, over the more questionable risks of backache, neurological sequelae and bladder dysfunction, opinion is divided. It can be impossible to persuade

179

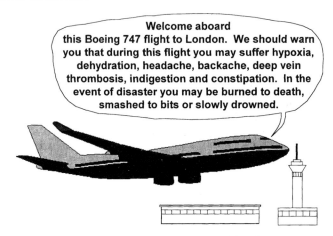

Welcome aboard this Boeing 747 flight to London. We should warn you that during this flight you may suffer hypoxia, dehydration, headache, backache, deep vein thrombosis, indigestion and constipation. In the event of disaster you may be burned to death, smashed to bits or slowly drowned.

There is no need to spell out every conceivable risk.

women, and some of their carers, that these are risks more of childbirth than of regional blockade.

The ideal time to discuss with prospective parents the role of regional analgesia and anaesthesia in childbirth is undoubtedly *before* labour. All too often anaesthetists are asked to provide regional analgesia in advanced labour when there has been no previous discussion of the pros and cons. Informed consent in such a situation, especially when the mother is under the influence of sedative drugs, is meaningless. The idea of antenatal education is, therefore, attractive but there are problems. Unfortunately those who most need antenatal education are the least likely to attend classes, moreover many women, especially those in their first pregnancy, do not consider that they will require regional analgesia and so do not wish to discuss the possible advantages and disadvantages. However, when in strong labour many of those with such antenatal reservations will ultimately request epidural analgesia.[3] It behoves those involved in antenatal education to try to reach all booked women and provide accurate information both on the need and the risks and benefits of regional techniques.

How to provide informed consent is another difficult area. In an ideal world each mother would be seen by an individual obstetric anaesthetist and her plans for labour analgesia discussed. However this is rarely practical and so other methods such as written information, videos and lectures have been used. It is extremely important that obstetric anaesthetists be involved in antenatal teaching about pain relief in labour.

When faced with a parturient in strong labour who has neither attended classes nor read books on pain relief, it is important to clarify that the attending midwife has explained regional analgesia to her, ideally in less stressful circumstances, and that together they have agreed to the procedure. Naturally this does not absolve the anaesthetist from all responsibility, but if the anaesthetist attempts to hold a protracted conversation with the mother, there is a risk of being told by the mother to "get on with it" – creating mutual animosity and a sense of guilt in the mother once she is pain-free. A desire by the anaesthetist to take written consent is merely an urge for self-protection, it serves no useful purpose for the mother. The midwife must document in the notes that the mother agrees to regional analgesia and it may be wise for the anaesthetist to sign these notes.

Preparation for regional analgesia

Anaesthetists should play an active part in the daily life of the delivery suite to keep up to date with the progress of mothers in labour. Thus when regional analgesia is requested the anaesthetist will be aware of any potential problems, and moreover appropriate tests will have already been performed so preventing unnecessary delay. The exact stage of labour will dictate the pre-block assessment and consent (see above). A mother in advanced labour who has lost control poses a very different challenge from one in early labour having only infrequent contractions. Whatever the situation, the anaesthetist must seek possible maternal and obstetric conditions that may alter anaesthetic management (see Chapter 8).

- The mother should have had her blood pressure checked no longer than 30 minutes before a block is established.
- The progress of labour should have been assessed by the attending midwife or obstetrician, and fetal heart rate should be monitored.
- A wide bore (16 gauge or larger) intravenous cannula must be sited. Despite claims to the contrary, this is painful and should always be preceded by subcutaneous infiltration of local anaesthetic.
- Insertion of the cannula may be a good time to take blood for full blood count, and group and save.
- Isotonic intravenous fluids, such as 0·9% saline or Hartmann's solution, should be given before labour analgesia. The infusion of a large amount of fluid is unnecessary and may lead to haemodilution and a resulting decrease in endogenous oxytocin secretion.[4]
- The partner or supporting person should be encouraged to remain present while the block is inserted to provide reassurance. The partner should be seated at the mother's head end so that communication and eye contact are maintained and also so that needle insertion cannot be observed, as this can make some feel faint.

181

Maternal position

When the anaesthetist has ensured that all the necessary equipment is available (see below), the mother must be helped to adopt the appropriate position for siting the epidural catheter. This is dictated by anaesthetic preference, maternal comfort, and the condition of the baby. Most anaesthetists prefer the mother to be either sitting or in the left lateral position. In either position it is necessary for the mother to flex the lumbar spine to open up the intervertebral spaces.

Contents of a regional block trolley

- IV fluids

- Giving sets

- Intravenous cannulae

- Needles

- Syringes

- Sterile epidural pack containing:
  drapes
  gauze for cleaning skin and for dressing the site
  gallipots
  sponge-holding forceps
  antiseptic solutions

- Epidural needles

- Spinal needles

- Loss of resistance syringes

- Epidural catheters and filters

- Antiseptic solution

- Adhesive tape

- Local anaesthetics (all ampoules should be sterile)

- Sterile sodium chloride 0·9% (some suppliers are willing to put this in the epidural pack)

- Ephedrine

- Blood sugar monitoring equipment (Dextrostix)

The **lateral** position may be preferable to the sitting as placental perfusion is better maintained,[5] although this has recently been challenged,[6] hypotension is less likely, it is more comfortable for the mother,[7] and monitoring of the fetal heart is easier. In the left lateral position, the mother's head but not shoulder should be supported on a pillow, to avoid any lateral neck flexion. Abduction of the lower shoulder should be avoided as this may distort the thoracic spine. Both shoulders should be hunched forward keeping the elbows together which keeps the trunk in a symmetrical position. The mother should then flex the lumbar spine. This may be done by telling her to try to touch her head with her knees. Excessive hip flexion can be uncomfortable and is not necessary if a mother is shown how to flex the lumbar spine by thrusting the pelvis forward. A sheet should cover the mother's bottom (but not her iliac crest) to make her feel less exposed (Figure 10.1).

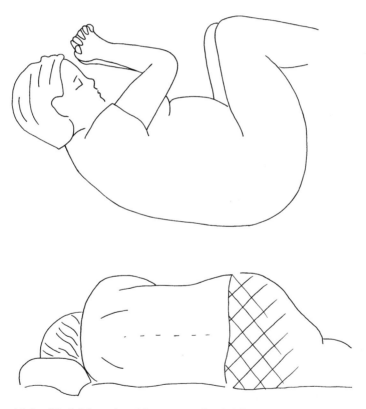

FIGURE 10.1—*The left lateral position, commonly used for epidural insertion. Note that the arms are together and well forward, the head (but not the shoulders) is supported on a pillow, so avoiding a lateral curve of the back. If the back is flexed at the waist as much as possible this obviates the need for excessive hip flexion, though this manoeuvre is often used nevertheless to force the back into flexion*

183

The **sitting** position may be preferred by and for the obese parturient and facilitates identification of the midline. The mother sits as far back on the bed as possible with her lower legs over the side of the bed and her feet resting on a stool. Her arms should rest across a pillow placed on her lap. Alternatively she may rest her arms on her partner who, provided he can cope, stands directly in front of her. She is encouraged to flex at the waist rather than the hips.

The anaesthetist should then don a face mask, scrub up and put on a gown and gloves. Gloves without starch are preferred as fibrous reaction within the epidural space may occur when powdered gloves are used.[8] The skin of the back should be cleaned with a suitable antiseptic such as chlorhexidine which should be given time to work while the anaesthetist prepares the equipment. This will take a few minutes and it is therefore important to reassure the mother and explain exactly what is happening. When all the equipment is ready, excess solution is wiped off to minimise the risk of its introduction into the epidural or subarachnoid space. Anatomical landmarks are identified. A line joining the two iliac crests (Tuffier's line) will usually cross the midline at the level of the spinous process of the 4th lumbar vertebra. With the increased lumbar lordosis of pregnancy, however, it may be slightly higher in the term parturient.

Epidural Analgesia

Equipment (Figure 10.2)

Needle A number of needles have been designed for epidural analgesia. The Tuohy needle is widely used in the UK. Available in 16 and 18 gauge, it usually has an 8 cm shaft marked at 1 cm intervals (Lee markings). It has a relatively blunt tip, angled at 20° (Huber point) to facilitate passage of a catheter. A wing attachment is available and is preferred by some to stabilise the needle during insertion. The Hustead needle, popular in North America, is of similar design.

Syringes The ideal syringe to detect loss of resistance is one in which the plunger moves freely within the barrel but the fit is nevertheless perfectly air-tight. Thus when the needle tip is within the ligament, pressure on the plunger advances the needle but does not cause the plunger to move within the barrel until the epidural space is entered. A good quality glass syringe fulfils this role best but contamination from glove powder may cause the plunger to stick. A specially made free-running disposable syringe (or loss of resistance device) is now included in many epidural kits and is preferred by some anaesthetists. Both loss of resistance devices and 10 ml glass

184

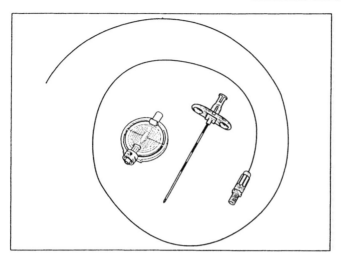

FIGURE 10.2—*The contents of an epidural minipack (Portex): details shown in* (a)–(c).

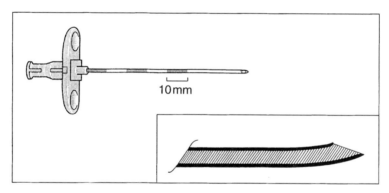

FIGURE 10.2—(a) *Tuohy needle, showing centimetre graduations and detachable wings; (inset) tip of needle.*

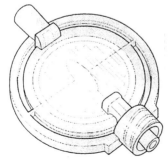

FIGURE 10.2—(b) *Epidural filter: an ideal two-way 0·2 µm flat filter, with female Luer lock to ensure that the catheter connector is firmly attached.*

185

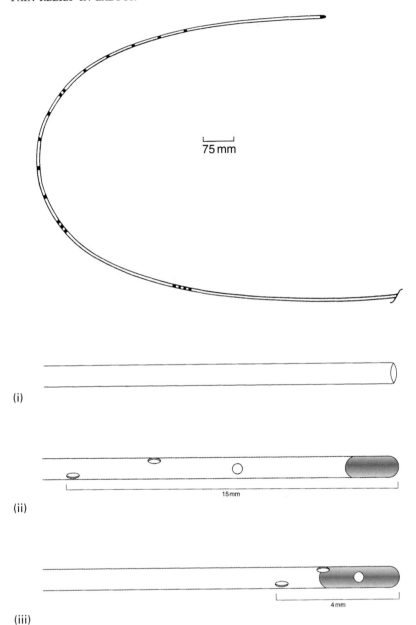

75 mm

(i)

15 mm

(ii)

4 mm

(iii)

FIGURE 10.2—(c) *Epidural catheter: (top) patient end, showing centimetre graduations with double mark at 10 cm and triple mark at 15 cm; (i) open ended, (ii) three helical holes, both distant (the original form) and (iii) closer, to minimise depositing solution in two different sites.*
Based on illustrations supplied courtesy of Portex

186

syringes may, however, have insufficient resistance to prevent movement of the plunger in the barrel before entry into the epidural space. Hence a 20 ml glass syringe or even an ordinary 10 ml plastic syringe may be considered superior.

Catheter In most situations a catheter is placed in the epidural space for continued drug administration. The catheter should be marked at intervals from the tip so that the amount of catheter in the epidural space is known. A catheter with a blind end with three lateral holes near the tip is to be preferred to those with just one terminal hole as analgesia is more evenly spread. Also the multiple side hole catheters are more likely to detect intravascular or intrathecal placement. Styletted catheters are available but are not recommended as insertion is associated with increased risk of nerve root damage and consequent prolonged paraesthesiae.[9]

Filter The outer end of the catheter should be attached to a 0·2 μm bacterial filter to minimise the risk of introducing infection. Should the filter become disconnected the catheter can no longer be regarded as sterile and should be removed. The filter also prevents injection of debris into the epidural space.

Technique

The mother should be positioned and the skin cleaned (see above). Before starting the procedure, the epidural equipment should be carefully checked and the catheter and filter primed with local anaesthetic. Local anaesthetic for skin infiltration is drawn up into a 2 or 5 ml syringe and injected using a 25 gauge needle. If sterile lignocaine is not available, in order to avoid drawing up local anaesthetic from an unsterile ampoule, bupivacaine from a sterile ampoule may be used for infiltration as it works equally quickly.

For pain relief in labour epidural catheters are best inserted at the L3–4 interspace. If placed higher, perineal pain may develop which is often difficult to relieve. The narrower L4–5 interspace can make identification of the epidural space difficult and spread of solutions to the lower thoracic roots is not reliable.

Various methods of detecting the epidural space have been described. The space may be approached from either the midline or by a paramedian approach and saline or air may be used to detect loss of resistance. For the midline approach the needle passes through skin, subcutaneous fat and three ligaments – supraspinous, interspinous, and ligamentum flavum. In the alternative paramedian technique the needle passes through the paravertebral muscles and then the ligamentum flavum.

The depth at which the epidural space is located depends on the mother's size, the interspace chosen, the approach used, the angle of needle insertion,

187

the technique for determining loss of resistance, and the degree of skin indentation.[10] The epidural space is furthest from the skin at L3–4 and the distance is usually between 4 and 6 cm,[11] although it may be as superficial as 2 cm and occasionally deeper than 9 cm. The depth correlates weakly with maternal weight and body mass index.[12] The distance which an epidural needle can be safely inserted before testing for loss of resistance has been investigated.[10] Dividing the woman's weight in kg by 25 gives the distance in centimetres at which the chance of accidental dural puncture is less than 1 in 200. Further advancement of the needle once the epidural space has been entered results in dural puncture at between 7·5 and 22·5 mm,[13] though off centre the depth of the epidural space may be negligible (see discussion of anatomy in Chapter 7).

In non-pregnant subjects there is usually a negative pressure in the epidural space. During pregnancy this pressure becomes positive and can rise further during uterine contractions.[14] Therefore negative pressure should not be used as a method to detect the epidural space in pregnant patients.

Midline approach (Figure 10.3)

Loss of resistance to saline With the mother suitably positioned, an interspace is identified if possible, preferably L3–4 (Figure 10.3a, b). Local anaesthetic is injected intradermally and subcutaneously. A small skin incision is sometimes made with a scalpel or Sise introducer to prevent drag by the skin on the needle. With modern disposable epidural needles, however, this extra step is unnecessary. The needle with stylet in situ is inserted in the midline, angled slightly cranially and with the bevel opening facing cephalad, the needle is advanced until gripped by ligament. The stylet is then removed and the saline-filled syringe attached. While the tip of the epidural needle remains within ligament, it can be advanced solely by steady pressure on the plunger with the right or dominant hand, while the other hand rests on the mother's back and holds the hub of the needle firmly (Figure 10.3c–e). A loss of resistance to injection signifies that the epidural space has been entered. Using this technique it is unnecessary to predict the depth of the epidural space, as the needle advances only while there is resistance to injection and stops automatically once resistance is lost – providing no sudden movement is allowed to occur. This is dependent on the resistance offered by the hand steadying the needle. The hand is braced against the mother's back, so moving with it. Needle advancement should be temporarily halted during uterine contractions. Sudden maternal movements and bulging of the dura increase the likelihood of inadvertent dural puncture whilst engorgement of epidural veins increases the potential for vessel puncture.

When loss of resistance has been detected, the syringe is disconnected. Injection of saline should be minimised to avoid confusion with CSF. A few drops of saline may drip from the hub of the epidural needle but rapidly the flow ceases and is readily distinguished therefore from the flow resulting from accidental dural puncture. Some practitioners have advocated introducing the epidural needle with the bevel facing laterally and rotating it through 90° upon entry to the space. This method is said to result in less damage to the dura and reduced incidence of headache in the event of accidental dural puncture. However, rotation of needles within the epidural space itself carries the risk of tearing the dura[15] and is not recommended. The aim of the technique should be to avoid dural puncture rather than to minimise the symptoms of its occurrence.

The catheter is then threaded down the needle so that ideally the 15 cm mark is level with the hub of the needle. More than this risks entanglement of the catheter; less and there may be insufficient in the space once the needle is withdrawn. For optimum analgesia 3·5–5 cm of epidural catheter should be left in the epidural space.[16] If 7 cm or more is inserted the tip may leave the epidural space through an intervertebral foramen, while insertion of less than 3 cm may leave the proximal side hole short of the epidural space.

On occasion the catheter may not pass easily through the end of the epidural needle. Once a catheter has been passed through the distal end of the epidural needle, however, it must never be withdrawn through the needle as there is a definite risk of shearing off the end of the catheter, leaving the distal fragment within the epidural space. If a catheter fails to pass easily it should not be forced, but may be rotated gently between finger and thumb; alternatively the hub of the needle may be gently pressed caudally or the mother asked to flex her back more. If these manoeuvres fail to allow the catheter to pass, the needle and catheter should be withdrawn together and the needle reinserted from scratch. Problems passing the catheter decrease with experience and may result from failure to keep the needle tip in the midline.

Once the catheter is in place the epidural needle is removed carefully so as to avoid withdrawing the catheter. Next gentle aspiration down the catheter will readily reveal if its tip is intravascular while continued aspiration of clear fluid may represent intrathecal placement. This may occur despite absence of CSF during needle insertion. It is unlikely that catheters can "migrate" from the epidural to the subarachnoid space when the dura is intact, since the catheter cannot penetrate an intact dura.[17] The thick dural membrane may, however, have been damaged by the needle, and insertion of the catheter may breach the much weaker arachnoid. Gentle aspiration down the catheter should continue while it is withdrawn to leave 4 cm in the epidural space.

An adhesive spray is first applied to the area surrounding skin puncture, and when this has become tacky a clear dressing is fixed. This may be helpful to assess inward or outward movement of the catheter during

189

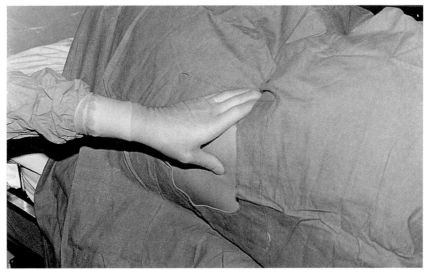

(a)

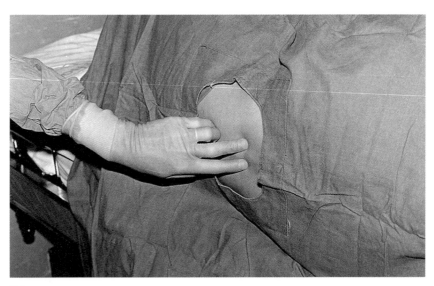

(b)

FIGURE 10.3—(*cont. over*) (a) *The fingers of the non-dominant hand locate the iliac crest and the thumb identifies an appropriate interspinous space.* (b) *The first two fingers then steady the skin on either side of the space in preparation for local infiltration (not shown). This should involve the minimum of prodding about. After infiltration, siting the needle, and removing the stylet, the loss-of-resistance syringe is attached. Pressure on the*

190

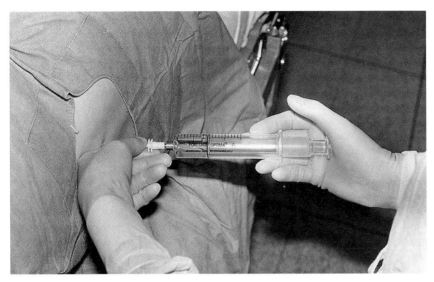

(c)

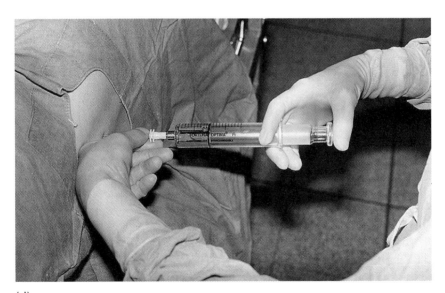

(d)

plunger may then be applied in one of three ways: (c) using the thenar eminence – the finger tips merely steady the barrel; (d) using the thiopentone injecting technique – possibly less sensitive; (e) (next page) using the true Doughty technique, in which some forward motion is applied to the barrel with the fingertips, while maintaining extra pressure on the plunger with the palm of the hand – possibly slightly less foolproof

191

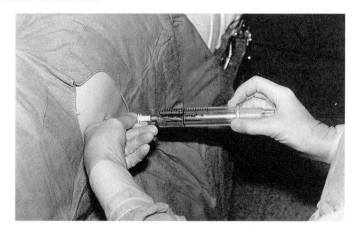

(e)

labour. The catheter is taped to the mother's back and over her shoulder permitting further top-ups to be given in a convenient position.

Loss of resistance to air   A different technique is required when air is used to identify the epidural space. Air in the syringe is compressible, and when the needle tip lies in the ligamentum flavum the pressed plunger will bounce back to its original position. The needle is advanced a millimetre at a time until air is injected easily, at which point the epidural space has been reached. The advantage of the air technique is that if fluid is seen in the epidural needle, it is likely to be CSF. It is preferable, however, to avoid dural puncture rather than to facilitate its diagnosis. Moreover, this argument is not foolproof, as previously injected local anaesthetic may track back in the needle. Disadvantages of the air technique are that it is slow, there is an increased risk of dural puncture,[18] an increased incidence of unblocked segments,[19] a risk of intrascapular pain if the mother is sitting, and risk of venous air embolus.

The paramedian approach

The mother is positioned as for the midline approach and the skin cleaned with antiseptic. The point of needle insertion is 1 cm lateral to the upper part of the spinous process below the desired interspace. Local anaesthetic is infiltrated down to the vertebral lamina. The epidural needle is inserted perpendicular to the skin and advanced through the paravertebral muscles until it strikes the vertebral lamina. The needle is redirected slightly cephalad and medially and "walked off" the lamina and into the ligamentum flavum.[20,21] Once in the ligamentum flavum, identification of the epidural space is either by air or saline, as for the midline approach.

192

Enthusiasts for the paramedian approach claim it is easier to learn[21] and has the advantage of more central catheter placement and less tendency to unilateral blockade.[22] The approach also produces less paraesthesiae with catheter insertion.[23] It is, however, a more painful technique, as the needle is walked off the vertebral lamina, stimulating the sensitive periosteum.[24]

Test doses

Detecting intrathecal placement

A dose of more than 15 mg of bupivacaine injected intrathecally would produce a very high spinal block. If a loading dose greater than 15 mg is to be given, it is therefore necessary to inject a portion of less than 15 mg through the catheter and wait to see the effect before giving the remainder. Subarachnoid placement is relatively easy to detect. Though 10 mg of bupivacaine has little immediate effect when administered epidurally, when given intrathecally it may cause sensory, motor, and autonomic block, resulting in labour analgesia, anaesthesia at S1 (a segment very resistant to epidural block), leg weakness, warm and dry feet (particularly the upper one) and possibly hypotension, within 5 minutes. When giving a test dose of small volume (2–4 ml), the nature of the solution used to prime the catheter and filter must be taken into account. If local anaesthetic has been used then a measured test dose of bupivacaine 10 mg will suffice; if primed with saline, then an extra 1 ml of local anaesthetic should be injected to allow for the fact that the first injected millilitre will be saline. It is not necessary to use lignocaine for the test dose as bupivacaine can serve this purpose satisfactorily.[25]

Detecting intravascular placement

Intravascular placement is more difficult to assess as a local anaesthetic test dose may have little systemic effect. The addition of 15 µg of adrenaline has been suggested to detect an intravascular catheter. However, the alleged rise in heart rate seen after intravascular injection of adrenaline lacks both sensitivity and specificity in labouring women, where heart rate changes are seen in response to pain.[26] Moreover, intravenous adrenaline may decrease uterine blood flow. Other suggested drugs for detecting intravascular placement are isoprenaline 5 µg, 2 ml lignocaine 5% and fentanyl 100 µg or even air.[27] There are, however, simpler and safer solutions to the problem.

The safest course of action is:

(1) Use a three-holed catheter, which is less likely to block.
(2) Observe the catheter for blood or CSF after insertion.
(3) Aspirate gently for blood or CSF before every injection.

(4) Inject extremely slowly while maintaining eye and verbal contact with the mother and looking for symptoms and signs of early systemic toxicity.

If the total amount of any bolus dose does not exceed 15 mg of bupivacaine, and it is injected *slowly*, then it may be argued that every dose is no more than a test dose. For example, 10 ml of 0·125% or 15 ml of 0·1% bupivacaine, each with 30–50 µg fentanyl, may be used as an epidural loading dose, but if inadvertently given either intrathecally or intravascularly should not result in either total spinal anaesthesia or systemic toxicity.

Loading doses

A wide variety of epidural loading doses have been used to achieve analgesia; most contain bupivacaine alone or in combination with other agents, most

TABLE 10.1—*Loading doses for epidural analgesia*

Loading dose	Comment
10 ml 0·25% bupivacaine 10 ml 0·25% bupivacaine + 1 in 200 000 adrenaline[30]	Increased motor block with adrenaline
10 ml 0·125% bupivacaine + 50 µg fentanyl 10–15 ml 0·1% bupivacaine + 50 µg fentanyl	Reduced motor block and increased maternal satisfaction compared to 0·25% bupivacaine
15 ml 0·04 bupivacaine + 25 µg fentanyl + 1 in 170 000 adrenaline[31]	Maternal ambulation possible
10 ml 0·125% bupivacaine + 5 µg sufentanil[32] 10–15 ml 0·1% bupivacaine + 5 µg sufentanil	Similar to fentanyl 50 µg
10 ml 0·0625% bupivacaine + 5 µg sufentanil[33]	
10 ml 0·125% bupivacaine + 25 mg pethidine[34]	
10 ml 0·25% bupivacaine + 2 mg butorphanol[35]	Possible maternal somnolence and fetal heart rate abnormalities
10 ml 0·25% bupivacaine + 5 mg diamorphine[36]	
10 ml 0·125% bupivacaine + 75 µg clonidine[37]	Reduced bupivacaine requirement in subsequent solution but increased maternal sedation compared to 0·25% bupivacaine

commonly opioids (Table 10.1). Opioids used as the sole agent may be effective in early labour if they are preceded by a local anaesthetic test dose, but do not produce reliable analgesia when given epidurally in advanced labour.[28] Many workers have added opioids to doses of local anaesthetics which are by themselves analgesic. Such practice is unnecessary as marginal improvements in pain relief are accompanied by side effects from opioid administration. Moreover, the potential for reducing the dose and side effects of local anaesthetics is lost.

The factors to be considered when deciding on an appropriate loading dose are the volume, concentration, and additives to local anaesthetic solutions.

Volume of solution To obtain appropriate spread to both lower thoracic and sacral roots when injecting at L3–4, the loading dose needs to be between 10 and 15 ml. Catheters placed at a higher level will require smaller volumes to produce analgesia at T11–12 but perineal pain from unblocked sacral roots may become a problem.

Concentration of local anaesthetic The concentration of local anaesthetic required depends on the stage of labour and the addition of other drugs (see table 10.1). Given in a volume of 20 ml, the ED_{95} of plain bupivacaine is calculated to be 0·129%.[29] As labour progresses, increasing concentration or opioid supplementation (see below) may be required. If given in sufficient volume a concentration stronger than 0·25% should not be needed, and incomplete analgesia suggests a misplaced catheter.

Supplementation The addition of opioids such as fentanyl to epidural solutions permits a reduction in the dose of local anaesthetic required to produce analgesia. Fentanyl 25–50 µg combined with 0·1–0·125% bupivacaine produces effective pain relief in early labour. As labour becomes more advanced increased concentration of both local anaesthetic and opioid may be required. The addition of diamorphine to the loading dose has been shown to improve the quality of a plain bupivacaine infusion.[36] Alpha agonists such as adrenaline and clonidine may also be used to permit a reduction in bupivacaine requirements. The addition of adrenaline, however, increases the incidence of maternal motor block,[30] while hypotension and sedation have been observed with clonidine.

Positioning

Following the test and/or loading dose the mother should be kept in the lateral position while the block develops. One of the simplest and most reliable signs of the onset of the block is an increase in foot skin temperature, particularly the plantar surface of the big toe. Often the lower foot warms more quickly or the mother is aware of decreased sensation on this side and it is therefore necessary to turn her onto her other side to ensure even spread.[38] In the absence of asymmetric signs, she should be turned to her other side after about 4–5 minutes. If the upper foot warms, this suggests the mother should not be turned. If abdominal pain is relieved but perineal

195

pain supervenes, then sitting her sloped 25° from the hips may favour sacral spread,[39] though sitting bolt upright may be counterproductive.[40]

When the mother is pain-free she may be permitted to sit upright, although her blood pressure should again be checked as this may provoke hypotension. Otherwise she should lie in either the left or right lateral position. **On no account should she adopt the supine position without adequate uterine displacement or a left pelvic tilt, as aorto-caval compression may result in significant impairment of placental blood flow.** For a further discussion of position and mobility in labour and guidance on maintenance of analgesia see Chapter 11.

Spinal analgesia

Despite its rapid onset of action, the place of spinal analgesia in obstetrics has been limited because it has usually been performed as a single-shot technique and analgesia does not usually last for the entirety of labour. It is therefore inappropriate for use in early labour, but it may be useful in advanced labour or for operative delivery. Also puncture of dura with the spinal needle during labour has until recently been associated with unacceptably high incidence of postdural puncture headache. Development in the design of spinal needles has reduced the incidence of headache.

Equipment

Spinal needles (Figure 10.4) The incidence of postdural puncture headache is directly proportional to the **size** of the hole in the dura, and so spinal needles should be of narrow gauge (24–29 gauge). However the ultrafine 29 gauge needles are technically difficult to use. With such fine-bore needles, CSF may not flow spontaneously from the needle hub and gentle aspiration may be necessary to confirm dural puncture.

Headache is also related to the design of the needle **tip.** Spinal needles are divided into those with a cutting point (Quincke) and those with an atraumatic tip (Whitacre, Sprotte) (Figure 10.4). The atraumatic tip appears to divide rather than cut the dural fibers, reducing the incidence of headache to less than 1%. Although the gauge of the Sprotte needle is relatively large, the bore is actually smaller than that of the B–D™ Whitacre, thus prolonging the time taken for CSF to flow from the needle hub. Another potential problem with the elongated distal aperture of the Sprotte is incomplete penetration of the dura. Although CSF may appear at the hub, not all of the solution injected reaches the subarachnoid space, producing an incomplete block. Improved needle design should take care of this problem.

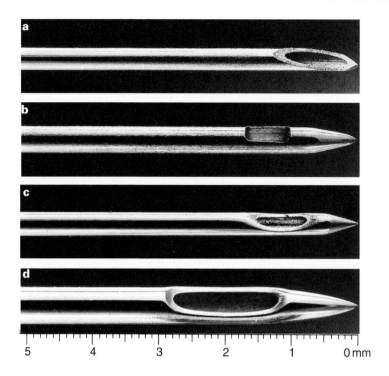

FIGURE 10.4—*Spinal needles.* (a) *Quincke point;* (b) *Whitacre;* (c) *Pencil point,* (d) *Sprotte. (Courtesy of Rusch)*

Spinal catheters Although atraumatic needles have been developed that allow the passage of a fine catheter into the subarachnoid space, doubt has been cast on their safety. The reason for this relates to the use of lignocaine, which unlike bupivacaine,[41,42] is irritant to nerves if allowed to pool in high concentration.[43,44] This is likely to happen when a hyperbaric solution is given to a mother sitting upright through a catheter whose tip is placed in the caudal part of the dural sac. Cases of cauda equina syndrome associated with the use of intrathecal lignocaine sometimes administered via microspinal catheters[43] prompted the FDA to withdraw the catheters, rather than hyperbaric lignocaine, from clinical practice in the USA.

Spread of spinal blockade

Several factors affect the spread of local anaesthetics in the CSF and thus the extent of the block. The most important of these factors are the baricity of injected solution, the patient posture and, to a lesser extent, the dose of drug.

Baricity Hyperbaric local anaesthetic solutions are those with a higher specific gravity than CSF, due to the addition of glucose. With the patient supine, hyperbaric solutions tend to produce a higher and more predictable spread than isobaric or hypobaric ones.[45] In the UK hyperbaric bupivacaine is used in nearly all spinal blocks.

Posture The spread of block produced by a hyperbaric solution is posture-dependent. Thus after a small dose (1 ml), block can be limited to the sacral roots (saddle block) if the mother remains sitting for a few minutes after an injection of heavy bupivacaine. This may be suitable for lift-out forceps or perineal repair. A block extending to the lower thoracic roots produces analgesia for any instrumental or assisted delivery and can be achieved by injection of a dose between 1·5 and 2 ml, with the mother in the lateral position with a slight head-up tilt. Immediately after injection the mother must be turned on to her other side to ensure bilateral spread.

Dose Increasing the dose may increase the height of the block, but its major effect is to increase the intensity and duration of the block.

Level To avoid damage to the spinal cord, spinal injection should not be performed above the L2–3 interspace. As this restricts injection to between L2–3 and L4–5, the level of injection is relatively unimportant.

Barbotage Repeated aspiration and injection is said to increase the spread of solution. However this technique is now little used as it may produce nerve damage.

Bevel The direction of the bevel or opening of the needle has little effect on the spread of solutions when other factors are taken into account.

Advantages and disadvantages of spinal analgesia

Advantages

(1) **Onset:** Spinal anaesthesia and analgesia have a more rapid onset of action than does epidural block.[46] Subarachnoid injection of bupivacaine and fentanyl produce analgesia within 5 minutes whilst labour pain may still be felt 20 minutes after epidural injection.
(2) **Quality:** A correctly placed injection produces a block of all adjacent nerve roots, including the sacral, with less possibility of patchy block.
(3) **Drug requirements:** Dose requirement for local anaesthetics is one-tenth that in the epidural space, which means there is no risk of systemic toxicity, even from accidental intravenous injection. Dose requirement for opioids varies less.

Disadvantages

(1) **Postdural puncture headache:** Until the introduction of atraumatic spinal needles, unacceptably high rates of headache limited the use of spinals in obstetric analgesia.

(2) **Technical difficulty:** The narrower the gauge of the spinal needle the more difficult it becomes to ensure correct placement leading to successful block.

(3) **Neurotoxicity:** Nerve irritation, arachnoiditis and nerve damage are difficult to produce by the epidural route, while there is a very real danger with spinal injection that drug errors, minor degrees of contamination, inappropriate formulations, and even lignocaine can cause nerve damage and may result in cauda equina syndrome.

(4) **Infection:** There have been reports of both infectious and aseptic meningitis following dural puncture in labour.[47,48]

Epidural and spinal blocks are compared in Table 10.2.

TABLE 10.2—*Comparison of epidural and spinal blocks*

	Epidural	Spinal
Onset of block	Up to 30 minutes	Within 5 minutes
Efficacy of block	Possibly incomplete	Usually complete
Drug requirement	Ten-fold higher than spinal	Small
Technique	Repeated top-up or infusion	Usually one shot
Headache	No headache without dural puncture	Headache related to needle size and design
Hypotension	Infrequent with low dose bupivacaine	More common than with epidural

Single-shot spinal analgesia

Single-shot spinal analgesia is most often used to provide blockade for operative vaginal delivery or for surgical removal of a retained placenta if an epidural catheter is not in place. In these situations surgical anaesthesia with dense motor block is achieved with local anaesthetic, e.g. 0·5% hyperbaric bupivacaine 2–2·5 ml. Rapid onset of autonomic block may produce significant hypotension.

Efforts have been made to find a means of producing spinal analgesia to last throughout labour by the use of morphine, diamorphine, and neostigmine (see below).

199

Intrathecal opioids (see also Chapter 7)

Fentanyl is often used with bupivacaine to provide spinal analgesia, though it has no product licence for this or for epidural use. A combination of 25 µg fentanyl with 2·5 mg bupivacaine produces analgesia lasting between 60 and 90 minutes.

Sufentanil is not available in the UK but studies from North America have demonstrated that a dose of 10 µg provides analgesia for between 1 and 2 hours.[49] Maternal hypotension has been observed in 11% receiving intrathecal sufentanil, and pruritus in more than 95%.[50] Higher doses increase the possibility of respiratory depression.

Pethidine has weak local anaesthetic properties and 10 mg injected intrathecally produces analgesia for about 2 hours.[51]

Morphine is slow in onset but has a long duration of action. The high incidence of side effects, such as pruritus, nausea, urinary retention, and drowsiness, limits its value.[52]

Diamorphine has perhaps been neglected as an agent for intrathecal analgesia in labour. Sneyd and Meyer-Witting showed that a dose of 2·5 mg could produce between 3 and 8 hours of pain relief with only minimal side effects.[53] A smaller dose than this has since been shown to be effective.[54]

Combined spinal epidural analgesia

Combined spinal epidural analgesia (CSE) has become popular for labour because it combines the rapid onset of spinal block, particularly valuable in late labour in multipara, and the flexibility of epidural techniques.

Technique

There are various ways to perform a CSE.

Two spaces; two needles The epidural catheter is sited first, followed by a spinal at a lower interspace. This technique was first described for caesarean section[55] but it may equally well be used in labour.

One space; needle through needle The epidural space is located with a Tuohy needle. A spinal needle, 9–11 mm longer than the epidural needle, is passed through it to penetrate the dura, and intrathecal injection performed. The spinal needle is withdrawn and a catheter is then introduced into the epidural space.[56] It is advantageous to have a spinal needle that can easily be held steady within the epidural needle. The technique requires practice, as problems may occur when initially attempted. The first problem is that the spinal needle fails to penetrate the arachnoid. This may be because the Tuohy needle has entered the very lateral part of the epidural space and thus the spinal needle cannot reach the dural sac. The spinal needle may occasionally pass through the dural sac and emerge on the other side. CSF may also fail to appear when the spinal needle is correctly positioned, as the distal opening may be occluded by the tightly packed cauda equina, or by an indented fold of arachnoid mater. A gentle cough by the mother, or rotating the spinal needle may help. Multiple attempts are not advisable. It is best to abandon the spinal and proceed to epidural analgesia. Another problem is that having administered the spinal, the epidural catheter fails to pass through the needle. This problem tends to disappear with experience. If it occurs, however, the epidural needle may be withdrawn, and if a hyperbaric solution has been given, the mother should be turned before reinserting it.

One space; spinal/epidural needle   The Tuohy needle has been modified for combined spinal epidural use. A double lumen allows the epidural catheter to be sited before the spinal needle is introduced. The equipment is expensive and not strictly necessary, as with practice the technique described above is satisfactory.

One space; two needles   Another modification of the single space approach avoids the need for special equipment or for hurry, as in the needle through needle method. An epidural needle is sited followed by a spinal introducer just caudad to it. After threading the epidural catheter, the epidural needle is removed and the spinal needle passed.[57]

Advantages and disadvantages

Advantages

(1) **Ambulation:** Using an intrathecal loading dose of 2·5 mg bupivacaine with 25 μg fentanyl followed by epidural top-ups of 0·1% bupivacaine with 2 μg/ml fentanyl, many mothers are able to ambulate during labour whilst pain-free.[58] Ambulation in labour without regional analgesia has been linked with a decrease in the length of labour, decrease in the need for analgesia, and an increase in spontaneous deliveries. However, at present such improvements have not been seen with ambulation during CSE.[46]

(2) **Speed of onset:** As the initial dose is given intrathecally, the onset of analgesia is far more rapid than with epidural analgesia alone.

(3) **Satisfaction:** When compared to epidural bolus doses of plain bupivacaine, CSE with low dose bupivacaine/fentanyl has been demonstrated to increase maternal satisfaction.[46] Increased satisfaction may result from rapidity of onset, short-lived motor block, and hence greater autonomy.

CSE is popular because it can produce rapid sensory analgesia without, in most cases, significant motor or autonomic block. As yet epidural techniques do not provide the same speed and degree of analgesia when ultra low doses of local anaesthetic have been used in an attempt to preserve motor function.[31]

Disadvantages

The disadvantages of CSE are essentially those of spinal analgesia.

(1) **Headache:** Using a 27 gauge Whitacre needle it would appear that headache is rare unless multiple attempts are made.
(2) **Infection:** Cases of both bacterial and chemical meningitis have been reported following CSE.[47,48]
(3) **Catheter position:** Concerns over forcing a relatively large epidural catheter through a tiny dural hole and into the subarachnoid space have been overstated.[59]
(4) **Failure:** A failure rate of 10% with the initial subarachnoid injection has been reported.[58]
(5) **Monitoring:** Continuous fetal heart rate monitoring by telemetry is required if women are to ambulate during labour.

Loading doses

The use of plain local anaesthetic to provide CSE[60] has been superseded by low dose bupivacaine/opioid regimens,[58] as the reduction in motor block

---

Loading doses for combined spinal epidural analgesia

- Bupivacaine 2·5 mg + fentanyl 25 μg[46]
- Sufentanil 10 μg[50]
- Bupivacaine 2·5 mg + sufentanil 10 μg[61]
- Pethidine 10 mg[62]
- Diamorphine 0·2–0·5 mg[54]

---

enables women to ambulate whilst pain-free. In the USA loading with sufentanil is popular either alone[50] or in combination with bupivacaine.[61] Intrathecal pethidine 10 mg has been reported to produce labour analgesia,[62] although it was associated with fetal heart rate abnormalities in 40% of cases. Diamorphine also provides excellent analgesia in doses of 0·2–0·5 mg but side effects of nausea, vomiting, and pruritus have been reported in 75% of mothers.[54]

Maintenance of analgesia after the initial spinal dose is similar to that for epidural analgesia and is described in Chapter 11. It should be remembered, however, that intravascular and intrathecal placement of the epidural catheter must be excluded by a suitable test dose (see page 193).

Other local anaesthetic techniques for labour

Caudal analgesia

The caudal approach to the epidural space was the first to be used to provide pain relief in labour.[63] However, because the dose required to reach T11/12 is so great, the quality of analgesia, especially in the first stage, is often poor, and the potential for side effects is greater than with lumbar epidural analgesia, this technique is now seldom used.

The caudal approach to the epidural space is via the sacrococcygeal membrane. The mother lies on her side and the insertion site is cleaned with antiseptic. The two sacral cornua which lie either side of the sacrococcygeal membrane are palpated. After subcutaneous infiltration with local anaesthetic, a needle is inserted at an angle of 70° to the skin and advanced until the sacrococcygeal membrane is pierced and the bony anterior wall of the sacral canal is reached. The needle is then redirected and advanced 1 cm up the canal. It must be remembered that the dural sac extends into the sacral canal, usually to the second sacral segment, and that advancing the needle further than 1 cm increases the possibility of dural puncture.

After careful aspiration for blood and CSF, 20 ml of 0·25% plain bupivacaine may be injected slowly to provide pain relief for labour. Alternatively, if a Tuohy needle has been used, a catheter may be threaded into the sacral canal. A test dose similar to that for lumbar epidural analgesia may be followed by top-ups. To produce sacral analgesia, for example for instrumental delivery, a smaller dose will suffice, though nowadays many prefer a spinal saddle block.

Advantages and disadvantages

The caudal approach offers few advantages over lumbar epidural analgesia. It may occasionally be justified when the lumbar approach is not possible, such as in severe scoliosis, or if sacral analgesia is the main objective. It has been suggested that dural puncture is less likely with the caudal approach to the epidural space. However, it should be remembered that the dural sac may be only 1·5 cm from the sacral hiatus.

The disadvantages are several:

(1) **Analgesia:** A block to the lower thoracic nerve roots is required for adequate first stage analgesia. Large volumes of local anaesthetic are

203

therefore necessary and result in perineal numbness and significant motor block of the legs.

(2) **Instrumental delivery:** The dense sensory block of the perineum may blunt the endogenous release of oxytocin in the second stage (Ferguson's reflex) and may impair the mother's ability to push effectively. Repeated doses given by the caudal route also produce a dense motor block of the pelvic floor muscles which may increase the incidence of malrotation.

(3) **Hypotension:** Autonomic block with resulting hypotension may follow caudal injection of local anaesthetic, though this should be less of a problem than with the lumbar route.

(3) **Local anaesthetic toxicity:** As large doses of local anaesthetic are required to provide adequate analgesia, the potential for drug toxicity is increased.

(4) **Variation in sacral anatomy:** This is common, and is the cause of a high failure rate for caudal analgesia. In some cases the sacral hiatus may be virtually non-existent and in others it may extend the entire length of the sacrum.

(5) **Infection:** Due to the close proximity of the anus, caudal analgesia carries a greater risk of infection, particularly if a catheter is inserted.

(6) **Fetal damage:** There have been case reports in which accidental injection into the fetal head has occurred during attempted caudal analgesia.[64] This not only damages the fetal head, it also causes life-threatening local anaesthetic toxicity.

As the disadvantages far outweigh any potential benefit, caudal analgesia is only recommended for use in labour when the lumbar approach is impossible, for example after lumbar spinal surgery.

Paracervical block

Pain transmission from the uterus may be blocked at the base of the broad ligament lateral to the cervix. Local anaesthetics injected at this site relieve the pain of the first stage of labour. A guarded needle is introduced into the lateral vaginal fornix and advanced 2–3 mm through the vaginal mucosa. After aspiration up to 10 ml of dilute local anaesthetic is injected and the procedure repeated on the opposite side.

Advantages and disadvantages

Although now rarely used in the UK because of the adverse effects, the technique has the advantage that it may be performed by the obstetrician, and for this reason it remains popular where anaesthetists are not routinely available, such as in parts of Scandinavia.[65,66]

The major adverse effect associated with paracervical block is the development of fetal bradycardia within 10 minutes of injection. Several theories for the bradycardia have been suggested, including direct local anaesthetic toxicity in the fetus,[67] reflex bradycardia from manipulation of the fetal head and that local anaesthetic produces uterine artery vasoconstriction with reduction of uteroplacental perfusion.

There is a possible danger of misplaced injection with a paracervical block. Injection into the uterine artery may produce fetal local anaesthetic toxicity whilst injection into the fetus will have similar effects and result in possible fetal death.

A paracervical block only relieves uterine contraction pain and lasts 90–210 minutes depending on which local anaesthetic is used. For outlet analgesia, pudendal nerve block (see below) is required in addition. The total dosage of local anaesthetic if the blocks are combined carries a significant risk of toxicity.

Pudendal block

The pudendal nerve carries sensation from the lower vagina, vulva, and perineum and the motor supply to the perineal muscles and the external anal sphincter. Pudendal nerve block has no effect on the pain of uterine contractions but it may be used for simple instrumental delivery where spinal or epidural blockade are unavailable or contraindicated.

Pudendal nerve block is almost always performed by an obstetrician. Either the transvaginal or transperineal approach may be used.

Transvaginal With the mother in the lithotomy position (ensuring adequate uterine displacement), a guarded needle is introduced through the side wall of the vagina and into the sacrospinous ligament, medial and posterior to the ischial spine. The needle is advanced until it emerges from the ligament and, following aspiration, 10 ml of 1% lignocaine is injected.

Transperineal This is the less reliable technique and is used only when the presenting part of the baby is too low to permit the transvaginal approach. The needle is inserted through the perineum at a point half way between the fourchette and the ischial tuberosity and advanced until the tip lies behind the ischial spine.

Infiltration of the perineum is usually performed in conjunction with pudendal block.

Pudendal nerve block has a high failure rate. Studies have reported successful bilateral block in only 50% of cases with the transvaginal approach and just 25% with the transperineal. Such poor performance may reflect lack of practice or waiting an insufficient time for the block to take effect.

Therefore if reliable analgesia is required spinal or epidural analgesia is preferable.

Complications of pudendal block are intravascular injection into the adjacent pudendal vessels, vaginal and ischiorectal haematoma, and retropsoal and subgluteal abscess.

References

1 Bogod D. What to tell the patient: consent and communication. (Abstract) Obstetric Anaesthetists' Association meeting, Basle, September 1995;pp53–4.
2 Bush DJ. A comparison of informed consent for obstetric anaesthesia in the USA and the UK. *Int J Obstet Anesth* 1995;4:1–6.
3 Rickford WJK, Reynolds F. Expectations and reality of labor pain and analgesia. Society of Obstetric Anesthetists and Perinatologists 19th Annual Meeting, Halifax, Nova Scotia 1987:163.
4 Cheek TG, Samuels P, Miller F, Tobin M, Gutsche BB. Normal saline i.v. fluid load decreases uterine activity in active labour. *Br J Anaesth* 1996;77:632–5.
5 Suonio S, Simpanen AL, Olkkonen H *et al.* Effect of left lateral recumbent position compare with supine and upright positions on placental blood in normal late pregnancy. *Ann Clin Res* 1976;8:22–6.
6 Chadwick IS, Eddleston JM, Candelier CK, Pollard BJ. Haemodynamic effects of the position chosen for the insertion of an epidural catheter. *Int J Obstet Anesth* 1993;2: 197–201.
7 Vincent RD, Chestnut DH. Which position is more comfortable for the parturient during identification of the epidural space? *Int J Obstet Anesth* 1991;1:9–11.
8 Green MA, Lam Y, Ross RF. Starch, gloves and epidural catheters. *Br J Anaesth* 1995; 75:768–70.
9 Yoshii WY, Rottman RL, Rosenblatt RM *et al.* Epidural catheter induced traumatic radiculopathy in obstetrics: one center's experience. *Reg Anesth* 1994;119:132–5.
10 Upton PM, Carrie LES, Reynolds K. Epidural insertion: how far should the epidural needle be inserted before testing for loss of resistance? *Int J Obstet Anesth* 1992;1:71–3.
11 Harrison GR, Clowes NWB. The depth of the lumbar epidural space from the skin. *Anaesthesia* 1985;40:685–7.
12 Meiklejohn BH. Distance from the skin to the lumbar epidural space in an obstetric population. *Reg Anesth* 1990;3:134–6.
13 Holloway TE, Telford R. Observations on deliberate dural puncture with a Tuohy needle. *Anaesthesia* 1991;46:722–4.
14 Messih MNA. Epidural space pressures in the lumbar region during pregnancy. *Anaesthesia* 1981;36:775.
15 Meiklejohn BH. The effect of rotation of an epidural needle: an in vitro study. *Anaesthesia* 1987;42:1180–2.
16 Beilin Y, Bernstein HH, Zucker-Pinchoff B. The optimal distance that a multiorifice epidural catheter should be threaded into the epidural space. *Anesth Analg* 1995;81:301–4.
17 Hardy PAJ. Can epidural catheters penetrate dura mater? An anatomical study. *Anaesthesia* 1986;41:1146–7.
18 Stride PC, Cooper GM. Dural taps revisited. A 20 year survey from the Birmingham Maternity Hospital. *Anaesthesia* 1993;48:247–55.
19 Valentine SJ, Jarvis AP, Shutt LE. Comparative study of the effects of air or saline to identify the extradural space. *Br J Anaesth* 1991;66:224–7.
20 Carrie LES. The approach to the extradural space. *Anaesthesia* 1971;26:252–3.
21 Carrie LES. The paramedian approach to the epidural space. *Anaesthesia* 1977;32:670–1.
22 Bloomberg RG. Technical advantages of the paramedian approach for lumbar epidural puncture and catheter introduction. *Anaesthesia* 1988;43:837–43.

23 Gaynor PA. The lumbar epidural region: anatomy and approach. In: Reynolds F, ed. *Epidural and spinal blockade in obstetrics*. London: Baillière Tindall, 1990:3–18.

24 Griffin RM, Scott RPF. A comparison between midline and paramedian approach to the extradural space. *Anaesthesia* 1984;**39**:584–6.

25 Reynolds F, Speedy HM. The subdural space: the third place to go astray. *Anaesthesia* 1990;**45**:120–3.

26 Leighton BL, Norris MC, Sosis M, Epstein R, Chayen B, Larijani GE. Limitations of epinephrine as a marker of intravascular injection in laboring women. *Anesthesiology* 1987; **66**:688–91.

27 Leighton BL, Norris MC, DeSimone CA. The air test as a clinically useful indicator of intravenously placed epidural catheters. *Anesthesiology* 1990;**73**:610–13.

28 Reynolds F, O'Sullivan G. Epidural fentanyl and perineal pain in labour. *Anaesthesia* 1989;**44**:341–4.

29 Columb MO, Lyons G. Determination of the minimum local analgesic concentration of epidural bupivacaine and lidocaine in labor. *Anesth Analg* 1995;**81**:833–7.

30 Yarnell RW, Ewing DA, Tierney E. Sacralization of epidural block with repeated doses of 0·25% bupivacaine during labor. *Reg Anesth* 1990;**15**:275–9.

31 Breen TW, Shapiro T, Glass B, Foster-Payne D, Oriol NE. Epidural anesthesia for labor in an ambulatory patient. *Anesth Analg* 1993;**77**:919–24.

32 Russell R, Groves P, Reynolds F. Is opioid loading necessary before opioid/local anaesthetic epidural infusions? *Int J Obstet Anesth* 1993;**2**:78–84.

33 Naulty JS. Epidural and spinal opiates in labour. In: Reynolds F, ed. *Epidural and spinal blockade in obstetrics*. London: Baillière Tindall, 1990:171–82.

34 Brownridge P, Plummer J, Mitchell J, Marshall P. An evaluation of epidural bupivacaine with and without meperidine in labor. *Reg Anesth* 1992;**17**:15–21.

35 Hunt CO, Naulty JS, Malinow AM, Datta S, Ostheimer GW. Epidural butorphanol-bupivacaine for analgesia during labor and delivery. *Anesth Analg* 1989;**68**:323–7.

36 McGrady EM, Brownhill DK, Davis AG. Epidural diamorphine and bupivacaine in labour. *Anaesthesia* 1989;**44**:400–3.

37 Brichant JF, Bonhomme V, Mikulski M, Lamy M, Hans P. Admixture of clonidine to extradural bupivacaine for analgesia during labor: effect of varying clonidine doses. *Anesthesiology* 1994;**81**:A1136.

38 Griffin R, Reynolds F. The association between foot temperature and asymmetrical epidural blockade. *Int J Obstet Anesth* 1994;**3**:132–6.

39 Griffin R, Barklamb M, Reynolds F. The effect of position on sacral spread of epidural analgesia. *Int J Obstet Anesth* 1994;**3**:31–4.

40 Merry AF, Cross JA, Mayadeo SV, Wild CJ. Posture and the spread of extradural analgesia in labour. *Br J Anaesth* 1983;**55**:303–6.

41 Hampl KF, Schneider MC, Ummenhofer W, Drewe J. Transient neurological symptoms after spinal anesthesia. *Anesth Analg* 1995;**81**:1148–53.

42 Tarkkila P, Huhtala J, Thominen M. Transient radicular irritation after spinal anaesthesia with hyperbaric 5% lignocaine. *Br J Anaesth* 1995;**74**:328–9.

43 Rigler ML, Drasner K. Distribution of catheter injected local anesthetic in a model of the subarachnoid space. *Anesthesiology* 1991;**75**:684–92.

44 Beardsley D, Halman S, Gantt R *et al.* Transient neurological deficit after spinal anesthesia: local anesthetic maldistribution with pencil point needles? *Anesth Analg* 1995;**81**:314–20.

45 Brown DT, Wildsmith JAW, Covino BG, Scott DB. Effect of baricity on spinal anaesthesia with amethocaine. *Br J Anaesth* 1980;**52**:589–96.

46 Collis RE, Davies DWL, Aveling W. Randomised comparison of combined spinal epidural and standard epidural analgesia in labour. *Lancet* 1995;**345**:1413–16.

47 Harding SA, Collis RE, Morgan BM. Meningitis after combined spinal-extradural anaesthesia in obstetrics. *Br J Anaesth* 1994;**73**:545–7.

48 Stallard N, Barry P. Another complication of combined extradural-subarachnoid technique. *Br J Anaesth* 1995:**75**:370–1.

49 Camann W, Denny R, Holby E, Datta S. A comparison of intrathecal, epidural and intravenous sufentanil for labor analgesia. *Anesthesiology* 1992;**77**:884–7.

50 Cohen SE, Cherry CH, Holbrook H, El Sayed YY, Gibson RN, Jaffe RA. Intrathecal sufentanil for labor analgesia–sensory changes, side effects and fetal heart rate changes. *Anesth Analg* 1993;**77**:1155–60.
51 Boreen S, Leighton BL, Kent H, Norris MC. Intrathecal morphine for labor analgesia: preliminary communication. *Int J Obstet Anesth* 1992;**1**:149–52.
52 Abboud TK, Shnider SM, Dailey PA et al. Intrathecal administration of hyperbaric morphine for the relief of pain in labour. *Br J Anaesth* 1984;**56**:1351–60.
53 Sneyd JR, Meyer-Witting M. Intrathecal diamorphine (heroin) for obstetric analgesia. *Int J Obstet Anesth* 1992;**1**:153–5.
54 Kestin I, Madden A, Mulvein J, Goodman N. Analgesia for labour and delivery using incremental diamorphine and bupivacaine via a 32 gauge intrathecal catheter. *Br J Anaesth* 1992;**68**:244–7.
55 Brownridge P. Epidural and subarachnoid analgesia for elective caesarean section. *Anaesthesia* 1981;**36**:70.
56 Carrie LES, O'Sulllivan GM. Subarachnoid bupivacaine 0·5% for caesarean section. *Eur J Anaesthesiol* 1984;**1**:275–83.
57 Turner MA, Reifenberg NA. Combined spinal epidural anaesthesia: the single space double-barrel technique. *Int J Obstet Anesth* 1995;**4**:158–60.
58 Collis RE, Baxandall ML, Srikantharajah ID, Edge G, Kadim MY, Morgan BM. Combined spinal epidural (CSE) analgesia: technique, management and outcome of 300 mothers. *Int J Obstet Anesth* 1994;**3**:75–81.
59 Abouliesh E, Rawal N, Shaw J, Lorenz T, Rashad MN. Intrathecal morphine 0·2 mg versus epidural bupivacaine 0·125% or their combination: effects on parturients. *Anesthesiology* 1991;**74**:711–16.
60 Stacey RGW, Watt S, Kadim MY, Morgan BM. Single space combined spinal extradural technique for analgesia in labour. *Br J Anaesth* 1993;**71**:499–502.
61 Campbell DC, Camann WR, Datta S. The addition of bupivacaine to intrathecal sufentanil for labor analgesia. *Anesth Analg* 1995;**81**:305–9.
62 Boreen S, Leighton BL, Kent H, Norris MC. Intrathecal meperidine for labor analgesia: preliminary communication. *Int J Obstet Anesth* 1992;**1**:149–52.
63 Hingson RA, Edwards WB. Continuous caudal anesthesia during labor and delivery. *Anesth Analg* 1942;**21**:301.
64 Finster M, Poppers PJ, Sinclair JC, Morishma HO, Daniel SS. Accidental intoxication of the fetus with local anesthetic drug during caudal anesthesia. *Am J Obstet Gynecol* 1965;**92**:922.
65 Kangas-Saarela T, Kangas-Karki K. Pain and pain relief in labour: parturients' experiences. *Int J Obstet Anesth* 1994;**3**:67–74.
66 Gerdin E, Cnattingius S. The use of obstetric analgesia in Sweden 1983–1986. *Br J Obstet Gynaecol* 1990;**97**:789–96.
67 Beazley JM, Taylor G, Reynolds F. Placental transfer of bupivacaine after paracervical block. *Obstet Gynecol* 1972;**39**:2–6.

11: Maintenance and monitoring

Maintenance
  Epidural analgesia
    Top-ups
    Continuous infusion
    Patient controlled epidural analgesia
  Spinal analgesia
    Continuous spinal infusion
Monitoring
  Contact with mother
  Sensory block
  Autonomic block
  Motor block
  Baby

Maintenance

Epidural analgesia

Intermittent bolus injection

The analgesic effects of the loading dose usually last between 60 and 90 minutes, although old-fashioned bolus doses containing 30–50 mg bupivacaine produce pain relief for up to 2 hours. Unless there have been complications, top-ups may be given by midwives who have been suitably trained in the management and complications of epidural analgesia. A checklist is of value (see Box). When using an intermittent technique, top-ups should be given as soon as the sensation of pain begins to return, as it takes several minutes for analgesia to be effective. Before a top-up is given it is wise to encourage the mother to pass urine. First there is more chance of the mother passing urine spontaneously when the block is not too dense, and secondly a full bladder may be the cause of pain despite a working epidural (see Chapter 12). The progress of labour should also be reviewed to check that delivery is not imminent, though it is inappropriate to delay pain relief while ritualistically carrying out a vaginal examination on every occasion. By and large a top-up would only be withheld if the

---

Checklist for midwife-administered epidural top-up

1 Check mother does not have a full bladder and encourage her to pass urine

2 Check progress of labour

3 Establish site of maximum discomfort and position mother lying on the least blocked side

4 Check intravenous cannula

5 Prepare and check appropriate top-up

6 Check epidural catheter and see that filter has remained firmly attached to it

7 Connect syringe to filter and aspirate gently for possible blood or CSF

8 Inject top-up slowly and observe mother closely for possible signs of local anaesthetic toxicity

9 Modify mother's position with any change in the site of her pain or asymmetry of foot temperature

10 Monitor mother's blood pressure every 5 minutes for next 20 minutes

11 If not pain-free in 20 minutes, call anaesthetist

---

head were visible on the perineum. After establishing the site of pain and positioning the mother appropriately, the intravenous line should be checked.

Before giving the top-up, the epidural catheter should be aspirated to check for blood or CSF. The top-up may then be given, injecting 10 ml over about 2 minutes, or in small divided doses. If the mother is not pain-free 20 minutes after a top-up, the anaesthetist should be called to assess the block.

As with loading doses, top-ups may contain various ingredients in different volumes and concentrations (see loading doses, Chapter 10). Bupivacaine is the local anaesthetic of choice and concentrations of 0·25%, or less when combined with opioids or adrenaline, are usually sufficient. Effective doses of 0·25% bupivacaine lead to increasing motor block if repeated.[1] Lower concentrations may be given but need to be supplemented with either adrenaline[2] or opioids such as fentanyl.[3]

Adequate volumes are required to ensure spread to both thoracic and sacral roots and 10 ml is usually required for each top-up when an intermittent bolus technique is used.

Top-ups are given as requested during the first stage of labour. In the passive part of the second stage before active pushing has started, a top-up should not be withheld as this will serve only to increase maternal distress without increasing the number of spontaneous deliveries.[4]

Continuous epidural infusion

Maintenance of epidural analgesia by continuous infusion has several advantages and disadvantages compared to intermittent top-ups.

Advantages

1 **Pain relief:** Using an intermittent technique, fluctuations in the quality of analgesia occur. At times pain relief is inadequate and at others excessive drug administration increases the potential for side effects. Such variations can be reduced by using a continuous infusion where the need for bolus administration is much reduced.[5]

2 **Safety:**

(i) Cardiovascular stability: Administration of bolus doses increases the risk of hypotension due to rapid onset of sympathetic blockade. By reducing the need for top-ups, infusions decrease the potential for hypotension and associated placental hypoperfusion.

(ii) Intrathecal injection: Should an epidural catheter lie partly in the subdural space and the arachnoid tears, total spinal anaesthesia may follow bolus injection. With an infusion the onset of symptoms and signs of spinal anaesthesia is gradual and should be spotted by careful monitoring before disaster occurs (see Monitoring).

(iii) Intravenous injection: As with intrathecal injection, the signs and symptoms of inadvertent intravenous drug administration may be detected in the early stages before they are severe.

(iv) Wrong injection: With a decreased requirement for top-ups the possibility for administering an inappropriate and potentially neurotoxic solution is reduced.

(v) Infection: The use of a continuous infusion reduces the need for catheter manipulation and accidental detachment of the filter, and may therefore decrease the potential for introducing infection.

3 **Workload:** Continuous epidural infusions can reduce the workload for both medical and midwifery staff.[6]

Disadvantages

1 **Motor block:** Initial studies of epidural infusions were performed using plain local anaesthetic solutions following a large loading dose. With such regimens, although the quality of analgesia was good, the incidence of motor block was high.[7] More recently, much lower doses of local anaesthetic combined with opioids have been used both for loading doses

211

and subsequent infusions. This has significantly reduced the incidence of motor block.[8]

2 **Equipment:** To set up an epidural infusion service infusion pumps and delivery tubing are required. The pump should be accurate, reliable and easily programmable. The advantages of continuous infusion should outweigh the financial constraints of purchasing such equipment. Nowadays pumps need not be cumbersome and indeed small versatile portable pumps, that can moreover be used for PCEA (see below), are available.

3 **Change in clinical practice:** Those involved in caring for women in labour may be reluctant to change their clinical practice. However, once the advantages of continuous infusions are apparent and adequate training has been undertaken this should no longer represent a problem.

4 **Feedback:** The spontaneous feedback provided by regression of blockade following a bolus dose is lacking. Hence careful monitoring is required to fine tune the infusion to suit the patient.

Before starting an infusion, an appropriate loading dose is required to render the mother pain-free. At this stage the spread of sensory block is documented and the infusion started. As with intermittent top-ups, there are many recipes for epidural infusions (see Table 11.1). Bupivacaine is

TABLE 11.1—*Epidural infusion regimens*

Contents	Rate (ml/h)
Bupivacaine 0·125%	12
Bupivacaine 0·1% + 2 µg/ml fentanyl	10
Bupivacaine 0·0625% + 2·5 µg/ml fentanyl	12
Bupivacaine 0·0625% + 0·25 µg/ml sufentanil	12
Bupivacaine 0·125% + 5 µg/ml alfentanil	10
Bupivacaine 0·125% + 25 µg/ml diamorphine	7·5
Bupivacaine 0·0625% + 50 µg/ml diamorphine	10

the preferred local anaesthetic for infusion, usually in combination with opioids. Lignocaine, by contrast, is more likely to accumulate to toxic levels in maternal tissues and to exhibit tachyphylaxis. Using an infusion rather than boluses does not alter this. To provide reliable analgesia by infusion throughout the first and second stages of labour a concentration of between 0·0625% and 0·1% bupivacaine is required. Fentanyl (2–2·5 µg/ml) is the most widely used opioid in the UK, although the successful use of sufentanil[9], alfentanil[10,11] and diamorphine[12-14] have all been reported.

Monitoring (see also p. 216) The severity and site of pain (if present) should be recorded hourly and in the event of supplementation. Maternal pulse and blood pressure should be recorded every 30 minutes. The height of block should be assessed by either ice or ethyl chloride spray at the start of the infusion, then every hour and after any additional top-up. The fetal heart rate should be monitored continuously during the infusion. Mothers should be encouraged to pass urine every 4 hours and when micturition is not possible catheterisation may be required to prevent over-distension of the bladder, leading to postpartum urinary dysfunction.

Analgesia is maintained by adjusting the infusion rate to provide an upper sensory level to T10. The usual starting rate for an infusion is 10–12 ml/h. If breakthrough pain occurs a top-up should be given and the infusion rate increased by 2 ml/h. Top-ups of 5 ml 0·25% bupivacaine are usually sufficient, although occasionally larger volumes may be required. Need for more than two supplementary top-ups suggests the epidural catheter should be resited.

If the sensory level extends above T10 the infusion rate may need to be reduced. If the block becomes dramatically more extensive and intense this could signal intrathecal infusion. This should be tested by aspiration down the filter and catheter.

Management of the second stage   The management of epidural infusions in the second stage should be dictated primarily by the mother's wishes, although guidance from an experienced midwife or anaesthetist should maximise the chance of spontaneous delivery. The height of the block and the degree of perineal sensation should be assessed and analgesia managed as outlined in Table 11.2.

TABLE 11.2—*Management of epidural infusions in the second stage*

Perineal sensation	Block above T10	Block below T10 No pain	Block below T10 pain
Present	Continue infusion	Continue infusion	If delivery not imminent, give bolus lying flat $\pm$ discontinue infusion
Absent	Stop infusion; reassess 20 min	Continue infusion	Give bolus lying flat and discontinue infusion

Patient controlled epidural analgesia

Somewhere between intermittent bolus doses and continuous infusion is patient controlled epidural analgesia (PCEA). PCEA doses are usually of smaller volume and given more frequently than traditional top-ups. The technique first described for labour in 1988[15] allows the mother to control her own pain relief with self-administered epidural top-ups with or without a background epidural infusion.

213

Advantages

1 **Autonomy:** Many women now want to participate more in their labour. By allowing maternal control, analgesia is titrated more to the mother's requirements, thus ideally avoiding periods of inadequate or excessive drug administration. Pain relief may even be withheld in the second stage if the mother so wishes. If and when bolus doses are required, they may be administered immediately by the mother.

2 **Patient satisfaction:** Many studies of PCEA have reported effective analgesia with high levels of maternal satisfaction.[16]

3 **Reduced bupivacaine dosage:** Some comparisons of continuous infusions with PCEA have demonstrated a reduction in total bupivacaine dosage without compromising analgesia.[16,17] Such reductions in bupivacaine have not been shown to reduce motor block or increase spontaneous delivery rate. However, it should be remembered that there are numerous PCEA and infusion regimens and no difference in bupivacaine dose has been demonstrated when PCEA has been compared to infusions of less than 0·1% bupivacaine with opioid.

Disadvantages

1 **Equipment** (see Continuous epidural infusions): PCEA pumps are more sophisticated and expensive than simple infusion pumps, although many modern portable pumps have PCA facilities. Pumps must be reliable, accurate, and easily programmable, and preferably small and portable.

2 **Anaesthetic input:** By allowing the mother to control her pain relief, there is a temptation for the anaesthetist to be less involved in her management.[18] Unlike intravenous PCA, where drowsiness limits further drug administration, incomplete analgesia from, say, a unilateral block may result in demands for repeated doses and consequently excessive motor block.[19] If PCEA is used it is therefore of the utmost importance that the attending anaesthetist should still play an active part in the mother's care.

PCEA regimens There are many different regimens that may be used to provide PCEA in labour, as detailed in the box.[20]

Early reports used bupivacaine solutions of either 0·25% or 0·125%, plain or with adrenaline. Although the quality of analgesia was good, the higher concentrations of bupivacaine tend to produce more motor block.[21] The use of 0·0625% bupivacaine with adrenaline and fentanyl has been demonstrated to be as effective as the higher concentrations.

The only opioids that have been assessed with PCEA are fentanyl and sufentanil. Fentanyl in doses from 1 to 3 µg/ml has been shown to be

PCEA settings for labour analgesia[20]

- Local anaesthetic bolus   Bupivacaine 2·5–5 mg

- Opioid bolus   Fentanyl 10–12·5 µg

- Bolus size   3–5 ml

- Lockout   10–15 min

- Background infusion   No advantage[22]

- Maximum dose/h   Bupivacaine 15 mg
      Fentanyl 30 µg

effective without demonstrable side effects on either mother or baby and, unlike its more expensive cousin sufentanil, it is available in the UK.

Most studies have used a bolus dose of 3–4 ml of solution containing between 4 and 6 mg bupivacaine with 10–12·5 µg fentanyl. Protocols should, however, not be too rigid and must allow for individual variation.

There is agreement that the most appropriate lockout time is between 10 and 15 minutes.

Using 0·125% bupivacaine with 3 µg/ml fentanyl, Paech found no advantage of adding a background infusion.[22] It is generally felt preferable for safety that no background infusion should be provided, but rather frequent boluses of small volume may be administered.

Monitoring   Monitoring should be similar to the procedures used with epidural infusions (see above).

Spinal analgesia

Continuous spinal analgesia

If a spinal catheter is used for continuous analgesia for labour, local anaesthetics and/or opioids may be used (see Chapter 10). Boluses of plain bupivacaine 0·25% 1–2 ml have been used, but a combination of 1 ml 0·25% bupivacaine with 25 µg of fentanyl produces rapid onset of analgesia with minimal and brief motor block. Intrathecal infusion of 0·125% bupivacaine has been used, but excessive motor block and low spontaneous delivery rates limit its routine use.[23]

One situation where continuous spinal analgesia may be indicated is following inadvertent dural puncture during epidural insertion. If an intrathecal catheter is inserted appropriate top-ups (bupivacaine 2·5 mg + fentanyl 25 µg) provide rapid onset of analgesia and, should operative delivery be required, surgical anaesthesia can be achieved swiftly and safely with 2 ml of hyperbaric bupivacaine. The alternative to a spinal catheter is to resite the epidural catheter at another space. Not only does this carry the risk of a second accidental dural puncture but top-ups given through the epidural catheter may produce a high block. This argument is discussed further under dural puncture (see Chapter 9).

Monitoring during regional analgesia in labour

Monitoring of sensory, motor and autonomic block is vital for successful management of regional analgesia.[24] After administering a test dose or loading dose, whether spinal or epidural, the anaesthetist should remain with the mother for at least 20 minutes, or longer should she not be pain-free.

Three to five minutes after a small dose, the following findings suggest intrathecal placement:

(1) rapid disappearance of labour pain;
(2) hypotension;
(3) motor block in the legs;
(4) loss of pain sensation on the outer side of the heel (the S1 root is resistant to epidural blockade);
(5) warm upper foot (plain bupivacaine solution is hypobaric to CSF but heavy in the epidural space).

During and after any bolus dose the following monitoring is required.

Contact with the mother

The anaesthetist should keep eye and verbal contact during and after any injection. Should intravascular injection of local anaesthetic occur the mother may report light-headedness, dizziness, circumoral tingling or numbness. Following unintentional intrathecal injection the mother may report numbness rising up her trunk, sometimes dizziness and nausea produced by hypotension, and difficulty in breathing before losing consciousness.

Sensory block

The most obvious sign of sensory block is the absence of pain during contractions. The upper dermatomal limit of the block should be assessed bilaterally 20–30 minutes after the loading dose and after all subsequent top-up injections. A blunted needle, ice or ethyl chloride spray may be used, starting at the inguinal ligament and working up gradually until pain or cold is experienced. It is necessary to allow sufficient time between stimuli for small nerve fibre conduction. Sacral block may also be tested, especially if perineal pain is experienced. This is most easily done by testing the back of the thigh (S2). Following intrathecal administration of local anaesthetic, the sacral roots are not missed. If an infusion technique is to be used, the upper limit of the block should be recorded at least once every hour and following any additional top-ups.

Autonomic block

One of the earliest signs of onset of an epidural block is an autonomic block producing warm, dry feet. Regular recording of whether both feet are warm and dry provides a useful objective index of symmetry and success of the block. However, of greater importance is the potential for hypotension with a reduction in placental perfusion. It is therefore mandatory to record the blood pressure every 5 minutes for 20 minutes after the loading dose and further top-ups, and half-hourly during infusions.

Motor block

Motor block is a dose-dependent side effect of the spinal and epidural use of local anaesthetics. Before ambulation, motor power must be tested assiduously. The mother should be able to raise the straight leg against strong resistance. Problems may be encountered on attempting to ambulate because of postural hypotension or from unsteadiness due to impaired proprioception. The mother herself may be able to predict her ability to ambulate. Assessment must be repeated after each top-up or at least hourly during the course of an infusion.

Baby

The fetal heart must be recorded before regional analgesia and this must be continued for at least 20 minutes after it has been instituted. Thereafter continuous fetal heart rate monitoring is preferable until delivery.

Pain

The site and severity of pain must be recorded before and after every top-up; similarly, during infusions breakthrough pain must be recorded.

It is not uncommon for an anaesthetist to be called to see a labouring mother because her epidural is not providing complete pain relief. The anaesthetist should first ask the mother where exactly she feels pain, when the last top-up was given, and what position the mother adopted after the top-up. This should be followed by an assessment of the spread of the block with ice or ethyl chloride. Foot temperature and sweating also indicate whether there is bilateral spread (see also Chapter 12).

Abdominal or back pain occurs if the upper lumbar and lower thoracic roots are not blocked. If an intermittent bolus regimen is used the return of abdominal or back pain implies that a further top-up is required. If pain is not relieved 20 minutes after topping up, an accurate assessment is required to determine the reason. Relief of pain on one side only with a warm, dry foot on that side may be the result of placing the epidural catheter off the midline or inappropriate positioning of the mother. When the block is tested by loss of temperature sensation, it is found to be absent on the painful side. Such unilateral blocks may be improved by further top-ups given with the mother lying on her unblocked side. Occasionally testing the spread of the block may reveal that one nerve root is not blocked, although those above and below are. Such a missed segment may follow the use of air to locate the epidural space or a bloody tap. A true missed segment is rare, however. Pain felt only in a small area on one side of the abdomen is much more likely to be due to the failure of the block to rise sufficiently high on that side.

Perineal pain is not uncommon as labour progresses and is the result of inadequate block of the sacral nerve roots. It is more likely to occur if the epidural catheter has been sited at L2–3 or above. Sacral spread of local anaesthetic solutions is encouraged by using a large volume and by placing the mother in a 25° head-up tilt,[25] but if this is unsuccessful in relieving pain, the addition of an opioid such as fentanyl to the top-up is more effective than local anaesthetic alone.[26]

The management of pain during epidural infusions is not dissimilar to that for intermittent top-ups, although the need for additional bolus doses is reduced. The mother's position should be adjusted from side to side according to the relative block heights on the two sides. By this ruse the incidence of breakthrough pain may be minimised. When pain occurs its site should be established and the extent of the block recorded. Top-ups should be given with the mother appropriately positioned and the rate of infusion increased. In most cases between 5 and 10 ml of 0·25% bupivacaine produces analgesia.

Where the dura has been damaged during epidural insertion it is possible to feed the catheter into the subdural space. A *subdural block* classically is slow in onset and may extend much higher than would be expected with epidural block, although there is often sparing of the sacral roots. The block is often patchy and motor block is minimal. If a subdural block is suspected the catheter should be removed as there is a danger of the arachnoid rupturing, producing total spinal anaesthesia.

(See also p. 232: *Record Keeping.*)

References

1 Yarnell RW, Ewing DA, Tierney E. Sacralization of epidural block with repeated doses of 0·25% bupivacaine during labor. *Reg Anesth* 1990;**15**:275–9.

2 Blayaert A, Soetens M, Vaes L, Van Steenberge AL, Van der Donck, A. Bupivacaine 0·125% in obstetric epidural analgesia; experience in 3000 cases. *Anesthesiology* 1979;**51**: 435–8.

3 Naulty JS. Epidural and spinal opiates in labour. In Reynolds F, ed. *Epidural and spinal blockade in obstetrics.* London, Baillière Tindall, 1990:171–82.

4 Phillips KC, Thomas TA. Second stage of labour with or without extradural analgesia. *Anaesthesia* 1983;**38**:972–6.

5 Lamont RF, Pinney D, Rodgers P, Bryant TN. Continuous versus intermittent epidural analgesia. *Anaesthesia* 1989;**44**:893–6.

6 Gaylard DG, Wilson IH, Balmer HGR. An epidural infusion technique for labour. *Anaesthesia* 1987;**43**:1098–101.

7 Bogod D, Rosen M, Rees GAD. Extradural infusion of 0·125% bupivacaine at 10 ml/h to women during labour. *Br J Anaesth* 1987;**59**;325–30.

8 Russell R, Reynolds F. Epidural infusion of low-dose bupivacaine and opioid in labour. Does reducing motor block increase the spontaneous delivery rate? *Anaesthesia* 1996;**51**: 266–73.

9 Russell R, Reynolds F. Epidural infusions for nulliparous women in labour: a randomized double blind comparison of fentanyl/bupivacaine with sufentanil/bupivacaine. *Anaesthesia* 1993;**48**:856–61.

10 Bader AM, Ray N, Datta S. Continuous epidural infusion of alfentanil and bupivacaine for labor and delivery. *Int J Obstet Anesth* 1992;**1**:187–90.

11 Hill DA, McCarthy G, Bali IM. Epidural infusion of alfentanil or diamorphine with bupivacaine in labour: a dose finding study. *Anaesthesia* 1995;**50**:415–9.

12 Enever GR, Noble HA, Kolditz D, Valentine S, Thomas TA. Epidural infusion of diamorphine with bupivacaine in labour: a comparison with fentanyl and bupivacaine. *Anaesthesia* 1991;**46**:169–73.

13 Bailey CR, Ruggier R, Findley IL. Diamorphine-bupivacaine mixture compared with plain bupivacaine for analgesia. *Br J Anaesth* 1994;**72**:58–61.

14 Lowson SM, Eggers KA, Warwick JP, Moore WJ, Thomas TA. Epidural infusions of bupivacaine and diamorphine in labour. *Anaesthesia* 1995;**50**:420–2.

15 Gambling DR, Yu P, Cole C, McMorland GH, Palmer L. A comparative study of patient controlled epidural analgesia (PCEA) and continuous infusion epidural analgesia (CIEA) during labour. *Can J Anaesth* 1988;**35**:249–54.

16 Gambling DR, McMorland GH, Yu P, Lazlo C. Comparison of patient controlled epidural analgesia and conventional "top-up" injections during labor. *Anesth Analg* 1990;**70**: 256–61.

17 Ferrante FM, Lu L, Jamison SB, Datta S. Patient controlled epidural analgesia; demand dosing. *Anesth Analg* 1991;**73**:547–52.

18 Eisenach JC. Patient controlled epidural analgesia during labor, or whose finger do you want on the button? *Int J Obstet Anesth* 1993;**2**:63–4.

19 Bogod D. Epidural infusions in labour should be abandoned in favour of patient controlled epidural analgesia. *Int J Obstet Anesth* 1996;**5**:59–63.

20 Paech MJ. Patient controlled analgesia in obstetrics. *Int J Obstet Anesth* 1996;**5**:115–25.

21 Paech MJ. Patient controlled epidural analgesia during labour: choice of solution. *Int J Obstet Anesth* 1993;**2**;65–72.

22 Paech MJ. Patient controlled epidural analgesia in labour – is a continuous infusion of benefit? *Anaesth Intens Care* 1992;**20**:15–20.

23 McHale S, Mitchell V, Howsam S, Carli F. Continuous subarachnoid infusion of 0·125% bupivacaine for analgesia in labour. *Br J Anaesth* 1992;**69**:634–36.

24 Obstetric Anaesthetists Association. Recommended minimum standards for obstetric anaesthesia services. *Int J Obstet Anesth* 1995;**4**:125–8.

25 Griffin R, Barklamb M, Reynolds F. The effect of position on sacral spread of epidural analgesia. *Int J Obstet Anesth* 1994;**3**:31–4.

26 Reynolds F, O'Sullivan G. Epidural fentanyl and perineal pain in labour. *Anaesthesia* 1989;**44**:341–4.

219

12: They think it's all over

It is not enough for an anaesthetist to be able to carry out practical procedures with skill, or even to achieve perfect regional analgesia swiftly; it is also necessary to ensure that analgesia continues throughout labour, and deal successfully with whatever problems may arise. Moreover, responsibilities do not end with the delivery of the baby.

Failure of the block to relieve pain

How do you assess an epidural block that is apparently not working or one in which pain is reported to recur? First, it is important to establish whether the block has *ever* worked, and to this end careful records throughout the duration of the block of the site and severity of pain, of block height, and of foot temperature are essential. In a perfect world it should never arise that a non-working block has been repeatedly topped up, but if this is the case and delivery is not imminent, it is best to fiddle about no further and to resite the catheter. If, on the other hand, the block has previously been working but the patient complains of pain, or if the initial dose has not produced satisfactory analgesia, then further assessment is needed and is summarised in Figure 12.1.

The anaesthetist called to a woman complaining of pain following epidural insertion, should, whilst greeting both her and the assembled

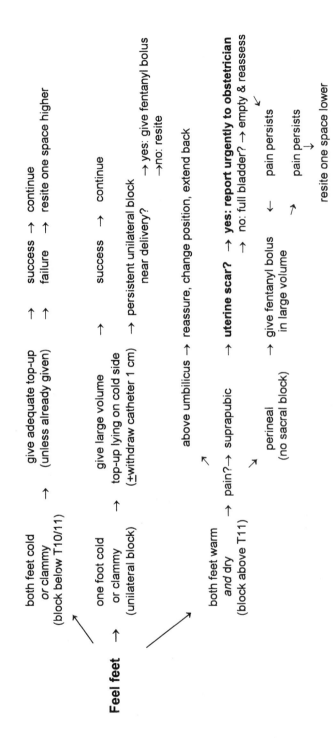

Feel feet →

both feet cold
or clammy
(block below T10/11)
→ give adequate top-up
(unless already given)
→ success → continue
→ failure → resite one space higher

one foot cold
or clammy
(unilateral block)
→ give large volume
top-up lying on cold side
(±withdraw catheter 1 cm)
→ success → continue
→ persistent unilateral block
near delivery? → yes: give fentanyl bolus
→no: resite

both feet warm
and dry
(block above T11)
→ pain? → above umbilicus → reassure, change position, extend back

→ suprapubic → uterine scar? → yes: report urgently to obstetrician
→ no: full bladder? → empty & reassess
→ pain persists

→ perineal
(no sacral block)
→ give fentanyl bolus
in large volume
↓
pain persists
→ resite one space lower

FIGURE 12.1—*How to assess an unsatisfactory epidural*

221

company, quietly feel both her feet (if she is still wearing socks then whoever sited the epidural has not assessed the mother properly). In the majority of cases a complete diagnosis can be made from this one brief act. Of course, in addition to feeling the feet you will also ask the mother where she feels the pain and make a careful assessment of the extent of block.

Interpreting your findings

Both feet are cold and clammy Either a top-up is needed or, if one has recently been given, this suggests the catheter has become dislodged or is sited too low. Test sensory block from L1 upwards. If no block can be detected even at L1 the catheter is *not* in the epidural space and must be resited. If a block is present but does not reach the umbilicus then try a large volume top-up with the mother horizontal or even head-down. If, however, a top-up of sufficient dose has already been given, it is preferable at this stage not to fiddle about any further but to resite the catheter one space higher.

One foot is cold, clammy or both The woman may need a large volume top-up lying with the cold foot down. If 4 cm or more of catheter have been threaded into the epidural space the success of such a top-up may possibly be enhanced by withdrawing the catheter 1 cm. If both these manoeuvres have been carried out without success, this constitutes a persistent unilateral block which has one of two possible causes:

(i) the catheter has gone straight into the lateral epidural or even the paravertebral space;[1]
(ii) the catheter may be in the subdural space.[2]

If the woman is too near to delivery for the epidural to be resited, it is reasonable to temporise by giving a bolus of fentanyl 75–100 µg with 10 mg of bupivacaine diluted to 10 ml (provided there are no contraindications). Since fentanyl works on the spinal cord, provided it can reach the subarachnoid space it should work bilaterally. If delivery is not imminent the catheter should be resited, making sure that it is not directed away from the painful side. After this, quite a small bolus dose can often achieve analgesia.

Both feet are warm and dry This usually signals a block of pinprick and temperature sensation to T10. The pain may be:

(i) upper abdominal, therefore not caused by uterine contraction – the mother may need to adjust her position, straighten her back etc.;
(ii) lower abdominal (suprapubic), but penetrating a functioning block;
(iii) conducted by the sacral roots.

With suprapubic pain the first question to ask is whether this patient has previously had a caesarean section or a myemectomy. A uterine scar *may* give rise to pain only during contractions. In the presence of a scarred uterus, suprapubic pain in association with warm, dry feet should be reported urgently to the obstetrician.

If there is no uterine pathology, the explanation may be a full bladder. The mother should be asked to empty it and then reassessed. If pain persists then it may be conducted by the sacral roots. Such pain is usually but not always interpreted as perineal. Test the centre back of the thighs (S2) as being easier and more humane than testing the perineum. If there is full sensation in this area this suggests the block is not extending low enough. Treat with a large-volume fentanyl bolus (see above) with a 20° head-up tilt *from the hips not the waist.* If this is unsuccessful and delivery is not imminent, the epidural should be resited one space lower.

After delivery

Once the placenta is removed, checked, and found to be complete, and provided there is no reason to anticipate severe postpartum pain (following caesarean section or major perineal trauma), the epidural catheter should be removed and checked for completeness. Occasionally difficulty is encountered in removing the catheter, in which case gentle traction should be applied while asking the mother to flex her spine. Usually adopting the position in which the catheter was sited will do the trick. Failing that, try different positions, even including extending the back.

Midwives have various rules about when a mother may mobilise after delivery. The time it takes for a mother to recover from the effects of regional block depends upon the dose of local anaesthetic she has received. In any case, the midwife should always tell the mother not to attempt to get out of bed unless an attendant is present. It would be normal to wait a few hours, then to assess motor power before allowing the mother to bear weight.

The postpartum visit

Any mother whom an anaesthetist has attended in labour should be visited in the postnatal period, not only to discover the fruits of the anaesthetist's labours but also to minimise the possibility that in his/her absence every minor postpartum ailment will be attributed to "the epidural".

When visiting the mother:
1) Congratulate her on her baby.
2) Enquire whether the analgesia was satisfactory. Enquire specifically about both first and second stages. Only thus will you learn whether

223

you have done a good job and whether you have instructed the midwives appropriately, or indeed whether they have been willing to carry out your wishes.

3) Audit her post partum symptoms

(i) Check that she has passed urine without difficulty. If there is any **hesitancy** recommend voiding while squatting down in a warm bath then quickly changing the water. It is amazing how often this simple remedy is overlooked. It easily overcomes the sort of hesitancy that commonly occurs postpartum and can, nine times out of ten, avoid the need for catheterisation. It is as important that the bladder is not allowed to become over-distended postpartum as intrapartum.

Next ask if she has any other complaints or aches and pains. The only one that may not be volunteered spontaneously is urinary dysfunction. For this reason, and because it must not be overlooked, it must be enquired about specifically. Other questions should be open-ended. The mother may report one or more of the following.

(ii) Primiparae may report **perineal pain**. It is useful to explain that this may be due to instrumental delivery, perineal trauma, stitches etc. Although many midwives will attribute this symptom to the epidural, there is no reason to do this. Perineal pain is less common among multipara, whether or not they have received regional analgesia.

(iii) Multiparae may, on the other hand, complain of **abdominal pain**, "after pains", due to uterine contractions. Again it is valuable to disclaim responsibility for this symptom.

(iv) If the mother complains of **back pain** establish whether this is local tenderness at the site of insertion or generalised backache. If the former, examine the site carefully and if there is no sign of inflammation reassure the mother that it will be better in a day or so. If there is swelling (which should be very rare), consider the possibility of local haematoma or infection. The latter may require antibiotics to prevent infection from tracking inwards to the epidural space. Take appropriate action and reassure the mother while inwardly castigating yourself.

If the mother complains of generalised backache or pain over the sacroiliac joints, explain that all this is due to the lax ligaments of pregnancy plus the stresses and strains of childbirth, not to the epidural. Give advice about back care and if possible ask the physiotherapist to visit and advise. For further information about postpartum backache see Chapter 9.

(v) The mother may mention **persistent weakness or numbness** in one or both legs. Occasionally a pocket of bupivacaine in a paravertebral space can have an effect persisting for 24 hours or so. If there is a history of unilateral block then this may well be the diagnosis. Examine the woman carefully, map the area of numbness accurately, and assess motor power round all joints. If there is the slightest suspicion that the block is not

224

resolving then an early neurological opinion should be sought (see Chapter 9, Neurological sequelae).

(vi) **Headache** is such an important complication it deserves a separate heading.

Headache

Headache is common in the days following delivery; it is therefore of crucial importance to establish whether a postpartum headache is due to dural puncture. The factors determining the incidence of postdural puncture headache are described in Chapter 9. Dural puncture headache is variable in site but typically postural. It is usually absent on waking but occurs when the mother sits up or ambulates and is relieved when she lies down. It may develop when she first mobilises, but commonly the onset is delayed until a day or two after delivery. Keeping a mother in bed after a known dural puncture tends to delay rather than prevent the onset of headache. A true dural puncture headache can occur after an apparently normal epidural,[2] which is why an accurate history of posture-related symptoms is so crucial. Occasionally, however, a mother may unconsciously adapt her history when she learns, from being repeatedly questioned, what symptoms are expected. If there is any doubt about the diagnosis apply the abdominal compression test. Sit the mother up and when she complains of headache grip her as tightly as possible round the waist (contraindicated after caesarean section). Do *not* tell her what to expect. A patient with a true dural puncture headache will report with surprise that her symptoms are relieved. Let go and they will recur. Advise immediate bed rest, preferably prone, and consider the next step.

It is a popular misconception that headache after dural puncture always resolves within a week. Regrettably this is not necessarily the case.[3] Headache may persist for months or years, may occasionally be associated with cranial nerve palsies, and is the commonest source of complaint following regional analgesia in obstetrics.[4] Moreover, when headache has been inadequately treated, cranial subdural haematoma and medullary and tentorial coning have all been reported, after either accidental puncture or even deliberate dural puncture using a small needle. In several cases failure to diagnose the condition resulted in death.[3]

Therefore, a dural puncture headache must not be neglected, and it is probably unwise to treat it symptomatically. Conservative treatment involving analgesics, caffeine, ACTH, drinking copious fluids, etc. is often advocated, but the danger is that this approach merely suppresses symptoms. The correct treatment must be to stop the leak and seal the hole.

To this end complete bed rest, which usually relieves the symptoms, must act by stopping the leak, and may be sufficient to allow the hole to seal itself following puncture with a fine spinal needle. If the headache is severe, persists for more than five days after puncture with a spinal needle, or if it develops after accidental dural puncture with an epidural needle, epidural blood patch is advisable. Autologous blood patch has a much higher success rate than epidural saline, and is the treatment of choice.

Epidural blood patching without tears

A woman who has a headache following accidental dural puncture is not only in pain, she is also likely to have little confidence in her carers. It is therefore essential that anyone providing an autologous blood patch must be competent and must also inspire confidence in the patient. Good stage managing is essential to preserve the patient's morale and trust. On the other hand, making a big issue of the procedure (referring to it as an operation, requiring special admission to the operating theatre, signing a consent form, etc.) can turn a mishap into a catastrophe in the mother's eyes. Blood patching literally at the bedside, provided that there is sufficient space, can make the procedure appear a suitably low key affair. Blood patching is contraindicated in the presence of bacteraemia, therefore some workers routinely send blood for culture before blood patching or at the time.

If, to minimise the apparent disturbance to the patient, it is thought appropriate to do a blood patch in a situation where epidurals are not habitually sited, it is doubly important to ensure that all the necessary equipment is assembled beforehand, as follows:

1 A second individual who is competent at withdrawing blood (ascertain his/her glove size).
2 A leakless sphygmomanometer.
3 A good size trolley with two shelves.
4 Two masks.
5 Two sterile gowns.
6 Two pairs of sterile gloves of the correct sizes.
7 Solution to clean the patient's skin.
8 Solution to scrub up with.
9 An epidural pack:
    and include: Tuohy needle
                loss-of-resistance device (glass syringe or other)
                small syringe for skin infiltration
                20 ml syringe for taking blood
                needle for skin infiltration
                needle for taking blood
                sufficient sterile drapes for both arm and back.
10 A nurse or further assistant.
11 Bottles for blood culture, if in the slightest doubt.

Before a blood patch procedure the woman must be apyrexial. She should rest horizontally for long enough to relieve her headache and, so that she feels relaxed, she should not have a full bladder. The optimum time to rest is therefore about 2 hours in case she has difficulty using a bed pan. The importance of complete rest is to minimise the volume of CSF within the epidural space, and so to avoid diluting the injected blood.

When all is ready, place the sphygmomanometer cuff with the tubing facing upwards as high as possible on the patient's *left* arm (if the *left* lateral position is to be used). After that help the patient into the lateral position on the edge of the bed (do not sit the patient up), position the pillow correctly to support the head but not the shoulder and ask the patient to keep her right arm out of the way above her head. Attach the sphygmomanometer to the cuff and position it out of the way. Make sure a nice vein is readily available.

Next the epiduralist dons a mask, scrubs and puts on gown and gloves; then the venepuncturist does the same. Meanwhile the epiduralist prepares the trolley, from which the venepuncturist may also work. The epiduralist cleans the skin of the back, applies a sterile towel and infiltrates the area as for a normal epidural. Blood extends cranially about twice as far as caudally,[5] so either the same space as the dural puncture or one lower should be used. The venepuncturist then prepares and drapes the arm so as to be able to keep the blood syringe absolutely sterile. A swab must be handy to press on the vein when the needle is withdrawn. When all is ready for the final approach to the epidural space, the blood pressure cuff is inflated by the second assistant to about 80 mmHg. The epidural needle is then sited using loss of resistance to saline, and 20 ml of blood is taken and passed across to the epiduralist while maintaining full asepsis. At this point blood may be taken for culture before deflating the cuff. When the epidural space is detected, minimal saline should be injected so as not to dilute the blood that is about to be injected. Provided the patient is adequately prepared, when the needle enters the epidural space very little cerebrospinal fluid should be present to drip back and cause concern. However, with a major rent there may be some drip-back of cerebrospinal fluid, but it will never be brisk. It is for this reason, however, that the epiduralist should be confident of avoiding a repeat dural puncture. Every step of the way the patient must be kept informed and encouraged to keep still. Patients are usually strongly motivated to do this.

With the needle in position the blood is injected slowly. During the course of injecting the blood the patient may experience discomfort in the legs or the back. Pause until the pain goes away and then resume injecting slowly. By this means try to inject as much as possible up to a maximum of 20 ml. When the injection is complete reattach the saline filled syringe and inject 0·5–1 ml of saline to clear the needle, to minimise back-tracking

227

of blood with the needle. Then remove the needle. Immediately apply a sterile adhesive dressing and turn the patient on her back. She should rest like this for at least 2 hours[6] then gradually mobilise while keeping her back straight. Instruct her not to bend her back or strain for one to two weeks. Encouraging her to be cautious in this way will minimise the chance of a recurrence of headache.

The increase in epidural pressure from the large volume of blood injected produces immediate relief of a postdural puncture headache, while the blood clot seals the dural hole. A stoical and sensible patient will experience relatively little discomfort from the administration of a blood patch but will usually report a remarkable relief of headache. Backache is common after blood patch but most women find it a fair exchange for the headache that they have been experiencing. Backache should disappear in a day or two.

Do not hesitate to repeat a blood patch if the headache has been relieved by the procedure but later recurs and is again a genuine postdural puncture headache. Blood injected into the epidural space is cleared from it remarkably quickly,[5] so does not hamper the success of any subsequent epidural block.

Once a patient is fully mobilised and free of headache, she may go home whenever she feels confident to do so. Remind her to avoid strenuous activity for a week or two and to keep her back straight when lifting and bathing the baby; this is a useful discipline for all to practise, as it minimises the chance of acquiring postural backache. Give her your telephone number and tell her to report to you if a spinal-type headache recurs, but reassure her that if she is careful it should not do so, and certainly will not after a few weeks. The community midwife should be familiar with the characteristics of a spinal headache, and can usefully assess the mother. It is important, however, that the mother does not lose too much confidence and does not come to attribute her every passing symptom to her mishap.

Teaching techniques for neuraxial blockade in labour

Who should teach?

Every consultant experienced in the art of neuraxial blockade in obstetrics should regard it as a prime responsibility to teach and train future generations of consultants. There is no case for trainees teaching one another, still less for the see one, do one, teach one approach in this field. The trainer must be experienced and confident and give the parturient and her partner confidence. Teaching is much harder than doing the job oneself, and in the same way that one gains experience in one's own practice, a consultant who is teaching practical techniques constantly and

228

conscientiously becomes a much better and more able teacher. He/she is better able to explain and give encouragement and to resist the temptation to take over.

A consultant must be responsible for seeing that every trainee is capable of carrying out the necessary techniques before performing solo. This should apply not only to novices but also to more senior trainees (see below).

Whom to teach?

It is sometimes stated that an anaesthetist should not learn to perform an epidural until confident that he or she can get out of trouble, for example able to intubate in the event of total spinal anaesthesia. This is surely a doctrine for the incompetent. It must be better to teach people how to stay out of trouble (Andrew Doughty, personal communication). Though currently in Britain it is fashionable to defer training in obstetric anaesthesia until the second year, a trainer who aims to maintain high standards may prefer to teach the young early in their careers rather than allow them to acquire bad habits in the operating theatre.

When to teach?

This is a hard one. How do you teach somebody to do their first epidural? Should their first experience be on an unconscious patient or on a model, or should they plunge straight in with a parturient? Though there may be a strong temptation to use an unconscious patient this temptation should be resisted. Siting an epidural catheter in an unconscious patient is undesirable at the best of times in that the patient can give no indication that the catheter is causing paraesthesiae or when needle or catheter is going off centre. A conscious patient is a useful guide to the midline. Also in some hospitals many more blocks are sited in the delivery suite than in the operating theatre. Hence the delivery suite offers the greatest scope for experience.

If on the other hand, a realistic model is available, this can be a good way to start, provided it does not engender over-confidence in the novice. Unlike a model, the human back is infinitely variable.

With the wide use of neuraxial block for caesarean section, the elective patient may be the ideal starting point for a trainee once a good demonstration has been observed. A teacher who is not confident, however, may easily find reasons why successive patients are not ideal for the trainee's first attempt. This one is in advanced labour, that one is too fat, a third may have a demanding partner, a fourth may be thought too distressed, etc., etc. Sooner or later, the novice has to take the plunge.

The progressive approach

The first stage in teaching is a demonstration. For this purpose a patient in advanced labour may not be ideal, as it is important for the teacher to go through all the procedures slowly, explaining every step of the way. The number of times that the trainee acts as an observer will depend upon circumstances, but once or twice may well be sufficient as there is no substitute for hands-on experience. In the next stage the teacher and the trainee scrub together and prepare the equipment. The trainee must learn to do this swiftly and with economy of effort. Each piece of equipment should be picked up and put down only once but everything should be ready for immediate use. The epiduralist must not have to break off in the middle, for example, because a syringe has not been loaded ready. Also unnecessary fiddling about is unfair on a parturient in strong labour.

For speed and to give the mother confidence it may be appropriate in the first combined effort for the teacher to prepare the equipment and to carry out the local infiltration. Not only is this swifter, it also means that the initial insertion of the Tuohy needle is less likely to be painful and so cause the mother to lose confidence. Thereafter the trainee may insert the needle under the close guidance of the teacher until the tip is held in the interspinous ligaments. The teacher should then remind the trainee exactly how his or her hands should be placed to ensure that pressure to advancement is applied on the plunger only and the non-dominant hand acts as a brake to a sudden advance of the needle. The trainee must be reminded how to brace the back of the non-dominant hand against the patient's back to this end. If when the trainee presses on the plunger there is no resistance to injection at the start of the approach then the teacher can immediately intervene to ensure that the tip of the Tuohy needle is squarely within the ligaments. The trainer then continues to make sure that the needle is correctly aligned and that slow but steady progress towards the epidural space is made. No jerking, twisting or screwing movements or intermittent advances of the needle should be made. Given an easy patient and a good trainee, he/she may soon experience the delicious and convincing sensation of loss of resistance, enormously enhancing confidence.

The trainee must be reminded not to inject excessive saline on gaining entry into the epidural space, he/she must be shown how to thread the catheter without force and without ever withdrawing it through the needle while avoiding contaminating it at any point throughout its length. (This may best be done by leaving the catheter end attached to a syringe on the trolley and picking up only the patient end of the catheter.) Once the catheter is appropriately threaded, the trainee must be shown how to withdraw the needle without also withdrawing the catheter, how to test it carefully, and how to adjust its position.

Trainees vary in the number of times they like to site an epidural catheter as a double act with a teacher, but gradually the good trainee will take over more and more of the procedure. The next step is for the trainee alone to scrub while the teacher remains in the room to act as an assistant, to ensure the mother's position is well maintained and to remind the trainee discreetly of any steps that may be forgotten. It is often appropriate for the teacher to appear to be present as an assistant and comforter of the mother while actually keeping a covert but close eye on the technical procedure.

Some trainees find this stage difficult and only blossom out when left alone. The first time this step is taken, however, the teacher must remain very near at hand and be ready to be called back quickly in the event of difficulty. If a trainee cannot find the epidural space it is important that the matter is put right swiftly before the mother suffers too long and becomes resentful.

A trainee who is well taught may never do an accidental dural puncture, but initially may have difficulty in finding the epidural space, particularly in obese individuals. Constant reassurance and confidence boosting are sometimes necessary to get past this hesitant stage.

After a trainee has been performing solo for a while it is necessary to go back and check up discreetly on progress and to make sure that no bad habits have been acquired.

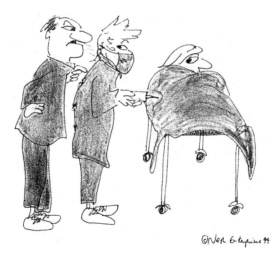

Some ways of checking up on progress can demoralise both doctor and patient.

Checking up on newcomers

In the training of young doctors in the UK, rotation is currently the name of the game, hence many young anaesthetists who have worked elsewhere with a variable and often unknown amount of training and supervision may come to work in an obstetric unit. It is the responsibility of the consultant in charge of obstetric anaesthesia to ensure that every newcomer is appropriately trained. Their skill or lack of it must not be regarded as a *fait accompli*, but must be assessed and if necessary tactfully improved. Some individuals at an advanced stage in their training are very happy and willing to receive further teaching; others, on the other hand – usually the less good ones – feel they have nothing to learn. In this case the tactful approach is to say perhaps that they still have to learn how to perform under a critical eye or how to teach.

Audit

Audit is fashionable in many contexts and it is particularly important in obstetric anaesthesia. Nevertheless it is a major undertaking to collect all the information that may be considered the absolute minimum necessary for adequate audit.

The consultant in charge of obstetric anaesthesia needs to know how all the individual members of the anaesthetic staff are performing, what their complication rates are and, in particular, whether accidental dural punctures have occurred. Any anaesthetist who experiences an accidental dural puncture needs to be debriefed and to analyse his/her technique in order to elucidate why the accident occurred and how to avoid it in future. Anaesthetists should look upon an accidental vessel puncture or dural puncture not as a chance event but as an error with a cause that can be analysed and avoided in future.

In order to keep prospective patients informed it is important to know how many women receive neuraxial block and what the complication rate is. Every unit should be able to quote its own accidental dural puncture rate, which should include typical spinal headaches after apparently normal epidural analgesia, since this type of headache is highly likely to require blood patch.

Hence in every obstetric unit it is valuable to collect, as an absolute minimum, the following information:

- How many epidurals, spinals, and combined spinal epidurals are performed for labour and how many for operative delivery
- What techniques are in use for detection of the epidural space
- How many accidental dural punctures and spinal headaches occur

Record keeping

Regional analgesia for labour requires immaculate record keeping. The process is complex and when pain relief fails it is impossible to sort out

EPIDURAL RECORD

Name: .... Age: ...... Para: ...... Date: .... CB: .... Last antenatal BP: ....

EPIDURAL TECHNIQUE

Space Used .... depth of epidural space .... cm   length of catheter in space .... cm

Indication: ....

Complications:

Dural tap:	none	needle	catheter
Bloody tap:	none	needle	catheter
Hypotension:	yes/no	treatment
Other (specify):		

Previous analgesia: ....

Opioid: ....

MAINTENANCE

Local Anaesthetic: ....

BOLUS	Test	load	2	3	4
Volume ml					
LA conc %					
Opioid µg					
Time					
Cx dilat cm					
Indication					
Signature					

INFUSIONS	1	2	3
Initial volume ml			
LA conc %			
Opioid conc µg/ml			
Start time			
Start rate ml/h			
Signature 1			
Signature 2			

FIGURE 12.2—(cont. opposite) *An example of an epidural record that is comprehensive and clear and yet will fit on to a single side of A4 paper*

INSTRUCTIONS TO MIDWIFE

Record:- baseline observations / changes after bolus / hourly assessments during infusions
Call anaesthetist if:- pain / 2nd stage / rising or falling block / severe motor block

													Anaesthetist (print name) ....
Time													
BP													
Infusion rate ml/h													
Block height (see over) — R / L													
Leg weakness None(0) Mild(M) Severe(S) — R / L													
Pain None(0) Mild(M) Severe(S) P = perineal — R / L / P													
Feet warm / dry / cold / wet — R / L													

Catheter removed: complete   yes/no   signature:

FOLLOW UP

Maternal opinion: 1st stage analgesia: Date: Delivery Type:
2nd stage analgesia: Onset of 2nd stage:
Satisfaction (0-10):   Time of delivery:

Perineal pain: yes/no   Headache: yes/no   Backache: yes/no   Bladder dysfunction: yes/no
Apgar score: 1 min   5 min

234

what has gone wrong without a full record of what has occurred. Equally, it is difficult to refute an allegation of negligence in the absence of a full contemporary record. Thus good records are particularly important in view of the ever-increasing frequency of litigation.

There are almost as many types of epidural record as there are consultant obstetric units. Yet very few of them make provision for all the necessary information, while many of those that do are several pages long. It is important that all the necessary information, including follow-up, can appear on one side of a sheet of paper. It is also important that forms are relatively easy to complete. If they appear too long or complex they are daunting and inhibiting. Periodic audit is required to ensure that forms are being completed properly and that patients are followed up postnatally. Figure 12.2 is an example of an epidural record that includes minimum patient data and details of the epidural siting, allows for a prescription separate from records of doses and infusions that are actually given, then records the outcome of the regional block on a temporal basis. This needs to include not only maternal blood pressure but also site and severity of pain or its absence, level of block, whether the feet are warm and dry and whether motor block is present. There is then space for a record of follow-up. Ideally these forms can be of self-carbon paper so that one copy remains in the patient's notes while the other can be kept in the anaesthetic department. On the back, a diagram of the relevant dermatomes can enable a midwife to record block height.

Complaints and litigation: how to minimise them

Regrettably, obstetric analgesia is now commonly the subject of complaint and threatened litigation. Women's expectations of childbirth have become so high that they may sue not only for genuine misfortunes but also because their obstetric experience and its outcome have not matched up to a preconceived standard of perfection. Although the latter type of complaint rarely becomes the subject of litigation, it frequently goes some way down the path and in so doing causes distress to all concerned.

Symptoms that most commonly form the basis of claims

- **Headache** This is the commonest complaint following regional analgesia in obstetrics[4] (see below and Chapter 9).
- **Backache** (see Chapter 9) Appropriate handling can prevent this symptom from being laid at the door of the anaesthetist.
- **Abdominal pain** This may follow a poor block and lack of rapport with the mother.

235

- **Baby problems** These are not often legitimately attributable to anaesthesia,[4] but if the anaesthetist does not form part of the team and fails to visit the patient postnatally then he/she may become the scapegoat.
- **Neurological sequelae**[7] (see Chapter 9) These are more likely to result from obstetric than anaesthetic problems[8] and early involvement of a neurologist is essential. The neurologist should be perceived by the mother as impartial and should also be able to make a more accurate diagnosis than the anaesthetist can. It is essential to make sure you can call upon a neurologist who understands that sequelae do not follow regional block out of the blue, that some cogent cause is necessary, and that obstetrics itself has its dangers.

It is important not to overlook the fact when dealing with neurological problems that peripheral nerve lesions may occur not only in the pelvis but also from peripheral compression (for example, the sciatic nerve in the buttock[9] or the perineal nerve at the head of the fibula). Make sure that midwives are educated to avoid such compression. Use a low dose local anaesthetic/opioid combination and make sure that the midwife knows that this epidural regimen should not result in complete numbness or motor block and that such symptoms should prompt a change of posture.

Quite apart from avoiding mistakes, negligent acts, and sins of omission there are many small things that can be done to minimise the chances of dissatisfaction and complaint by mothers. There is a common theme running through many stories.[10]

Common causes of dissatisfaction

Lack of information and consent

This often forms part of a complaint against an obstetric anaesthetist. Women commonly say, "If I'd known this was going to happen, I would never have consented." This sort of complaint usually relates to a symptom that the anaesthetist with all the time in the world would not have mentioned since it is unlikely to have been caused by the regional block. Few women who have attended antenatal classes and have obtained all the appropriate information do actually sue. Women who complain have frequently approached labour with a negative attitude to epidural analgesia and have only agreed to it when the situation has become desperate – way past the point where they want to listen to a prolonged explanation or can give it their attention.

Delay in obtaining an anaesthetist

This is, of course, more likely to occur in small centres where there is no adequate provision for a full epidural service. Care may thus not appear to be expert and streamlined.

What's in a name?

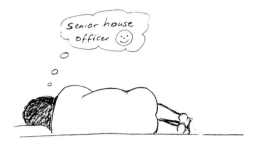

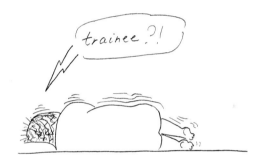

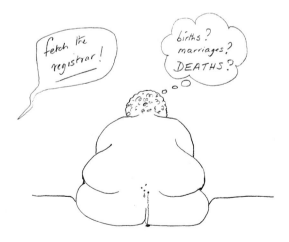

Lack of confidence in the anaesthetist

Everything possible should be done to enhance the mother's confidence in the anaesthetist. How other staff refer to the anaesthetist can have as effect on the mother's confidence. Also if the anaesthetist appears rushed and flustered the confidence of the mother or her partner will be undermined. The outcome of this scenario is likely to be that any problem that arises, big or small, may be laid at the door of this hard-pressed doctor.

Pain on siting the spinal or epidural

A nervous mother may react strongly to the simple process of infiltrating the skin with local anaesthetic and more still to paraesthesiae caused by catheter insertion, particularly if she is not warned beforehand. Such paraesthesiae are occasionally followed by an area of numbness or shooting pains in the leg postpartum. One must assume that damage to a nerve root may be so caused, particularly with a spinal needle. It is becoming apparent that mothers should be informed of this possibility before a regional block is administered. Occasionally, a mother complains of the most excruciating pain during the procedure, and this has, in the courts, been attributed variously to injection into the spinal cord itself (which would in general imply an anatomical abnormality, or a gross error in approach, the latter only being negligent) or to injection of a noxious substance. It is not necessary for the plaintiff to prove in court what that substance might have been in order to be awarded damages.

Unsatisfactory block

A mother may complain with one breath that she never wanted epidural analgesia in labour and with the next that it did not work anyway. The callous might maintain that such a woman has no claim, since she experienced the labour pain she desired. Nevertheless, such a situation is an obvious cause of dissatisfaction. Unsatisfactory blocks for surgery are of course a much bigger problem and currently a common subject of litigation.[4,10]

Failure to visit the mother post partum

A sympathetic and kindly visit, particularly if there is any reason to suppose a problem might have been caused (typically a headache), can help to keep the mother on your side. If, in particular, there is a headache, prompt and effective management by the anaesthetist is absolutely essential.

The moral is ...

- Do not attempt to provide an epidural service where manpower is inadequate.

- See that written information about pain relief in labour is given to every woman who books for delivery in the unit. This way the onus is on the mother to read the information. Although antenatal classes may be provided, the concern here is more with those who do not attend them.
- No matter how rushed and flustered you may feel when you attend the parturient, put on a calm and unhurried air. Be charming and polite to her and her partner at all times, even if they are rude and uncooperative.
- Decide how much information you think it is appropriate to give the mother. Satisfy yourself that the midwife has obtained verbal consent and written this in the notes.
- Warn the mother about the pain of local anaesthetic infiltration and of the possibility of paraesthesiae when you thread in the epidural catheter.
- Make certain that you achieve satisfactory analgesia during labour. After siting a regional block never leave a mother before she is pain-free. Visit her during the course of labour and make sure the midwife knows that you would like to be called if pain relief is unsatisfactory.
- Visit the mother in the postnatal ward afterwards (see pp. 220 *et seq.*).

AND

Avoid actual mistakes

Accidental dural puncture

Accidental dural puncture rates should always be audited. It is essential to know and inform prospective mothers of the local dural puncture rate. Every anaesthetist who is destined to take part in the obstetric anaesthesia service should be properly trained and assessed before being allowed to work unsupervised. With careful teaching and use of an appropriate epidural technique it is possible to achieve an accidental dural puncture rate, even among trainees, of considerably less than 1%.[3]

Adequate warning and an appropriately handled dural puncture should not lead to problems, but failure to make a proper diagnosis, to manage the patient correctly and to apply a blood patch efficiently can lead to endless problems for the mother in the postnatal period. Consequently she feels resentment towards the anaesthetist. Inappropriate handling of a postdural puncture headache sometimes results in a chronic headache even in the absence of a persistent leak. This problem is not limited to hysterics.

To puncture the dura accidentally *per se* has not hitherto been considered negligent, though failure to warn of the possibility and to attend the mother and offer appropriate care postnatally may be.

Wrong injection

It cannot be emphasised too frequently how important it is to use the appropriate drugs and to check them carefully. This is particularly vital for

239

subarachnoid injection, where it is so easy to do damage. Having two people check ampoules is a sensible nursing/midwifery practice that anaesthetists could do well to emulate. Errors do occur, and are considered negligent.

Wrong place

When one is tired and rushed lapses in concentration can occasionally result in intravenous drugs being given epidurally and vice versa. Nevertheless, even when such crass and obvious errors have occurred, honest and sympathetic handling of the woman and her partner ease the situation. If lasting damage occurs such a mistake is, of course, indefensible. Whether an accidental total spinal constitutes negligence, however, would be open to debate.

Keep immaculate records

Cases arise where a plaintiff who has suffered harm is awarded damages despite the absence of any real evidence of negligence, simply because the case notes are incomplete. It is therefore mandatory to keep careful and complete contemporary records. If anything does go wrong, write a full account in the notes as soon as possible after the event while it is fresh in your mind. When, therefore, a claim for negligence is made you can prepare a reliable witness statement with reference to both contemporary records and your own early memory of the case.

And finally ...

There is a long road between a complaint by a dissatisfied patient and a case actually coming to court, and thankfully only a tiny minority of cases reach the end of that road. Along the way, however, the process is unpleasant for all concerned and also expensive, whether in the end the plaintiff wins or loses her case.

If harm occurs, do not try to cover up errors. Be frank. Be prepared to explain to the patient, and to apologise if appropriate.

References

1 Collier CB. Why obstetric epidurals fail: a study of epidurograms. *Int J Obstet Anesth* 1996;5:19–31.
2 Reynolds F, Speedy H. The subdural space; the third place to go astray. *Anaesthesia* 1990; 45:120–3.
3 Reynolds F. Dural puncture and headache. Avoid the first but treat the second. *Br J Med* 1993;306:874–6.
4 Chadwick HS. An analysis of obstetric anesthesia cases from the American Society of Anesthesiologists closed claims project database. *Int J Obstet Anesth* 1996;5:258–63.

5 Beards SC, Jackson A, Griffiths AG, Horsman EL. Magnetic resonance imaging of extradural blood patches; appearances from 30min to 18h. *Br J Anaesth* 1993;**71**:182–8.
6 Martin R, Jourdain S, Clairoux M, Tétrault JP. Duration of decubitus position after epidural blood patch. *Can J Anaesth* 1994;**41**:23–5.
7 Reynolds F. Maternal sequelae of childbirth. *Br J Anaesth* 1995;**75**:515–7.
8 Holdcroft A, Gibberd FB, Hargrove RL, Hawkins DF, Dellaportas CI. Neurological complications associated with pregnancy. *Br J Anaesth* 1995;**75**:522–6.
9 Silva M, Mallinson C, Reynolds F. Sciatic nerve palsy following childbirth. *Anaesthesia* 1996;**51**:1144–8.
10 Reynolds F. Litigation in obstetric regional anaesthesia. In Van Zundert A, ed. *Highlights in pain therapy and regional anaesthesia, V.* Barcelona: Publicidad Permanyer, 1996:39–43.

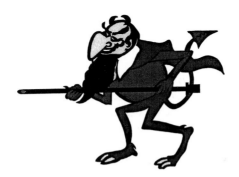

Index

effect
central nervous system 96
fetus 98–100
gastrointestinal tract, 96–7
labour 97–8
maternal respiratory effects 97
mother 96–7
neonatal effects 100–1
neonatal respiratory
depression 100
efficacy 93–5
vs nitrous oxide 9
vs other systemic opioids 94
clinical trials 94
pain score before and after 53
epidural analgesia 194, 202, 212
fate 91
frequency of use in UK 9, 93
late effects 101
loading doses for combined
spinal–epidural analgesia 202
maternal opinion 9
nausea and vomiting 96
pain intensity and sedation
scores 94
pharmacological
properties 90–1 133
physicochemical properties 90–1
ranitidine and metoclopramide co-
administration 97
routes and modes of systemic
administration 102–3
sedation *vs* analgesia 4
in spinal analgesia 200
structural formula 90
physical methods, management of
labour pain 36–58
physiotherapy techniques 19–20
placenta
retained, regional analgesia 141, 144
separation
and discontinuation of
oxygenation, 52
water birth contraindications 147
placenta percreta/accreta,
contraindications to regional
analgesia 147
placenta praevia 147
water birth contraindications 49
pollution, inhalational analgesia 81–2
postpartum visit 223–5

pre-eclampsia and pregnancy-induced
hypertension 138
pethidine contraindications 102
water baths contraindications 49
prematurity, indication for regional
analgesia 140
"prepared childbirth" 19, 25
pressure sores, and regional block 160
prilocaine
anaphylactic reactions 147
pharmacology 130–1
pro-opiomelanocortin 154
procaine hydrochloride
intradermal "anaesthesia" 53–4
pain relief 53–4
promazine, with pethidine 94
promethazine 164
proprioception, spinal–epidural
analgesia 153
pruritus, morphine 132
psychological methods of
analgesia 17–25
mechanism of action 20–1
psychological disadvantages 24
psychoprophylaxis 18–21
pudendal block 205–6
transperineal 205–6
transvaginal 205
pulmonary aspiration *see* aspiration of
gastric contents
pulmonary hypertension 139

Quincke needle 196, 197

ranitidine, co-administered with
pethidine 97
Read, Grantly Dick, "natural
childbirth" 9, 18–20
record-keeping, epidural
analgesia 233–4, 240
regional analgesia 120–241
autonomic block 153, 217
caesarean section 142–3, 163–4
coagulation disorders 144–5
contraindications 144–8
effect on labour and delivery 162–5
effects on fetus 168–73
fetal indications 140–1
indications 137–44
instrumental delivery
association 165–8